Update on Biomarkers in Allergy and Asthma

Guest Editor

ROHIT K. KATIAL, MD

IMMUNOLOGY AND ALLERGY CLINICS OF NORTH AMERICA

www.immunology.theclinics.com

Consulting Editor
RAFEUL ALAM, MD, PhD

August 2012 • Volume 32 • Number 3

SAUNDERS an imprint of ELSEVIER, Inc.

W.B. SAUNDERS COMPANY

A Division of Elsevier Inc.

1600 John F. Kennedy Blvd., • Suite 1800 • Philadelphia, PA 19103-2899.

http://www.theclinics.com

IMMUNOLOGY AND ALLERGY CLINICS OF NORTH AMERICA Volume 32, Number 3

August 2012 ISSN 0889-8561, ISBN-13: 978-1-4557-5091-7

Editor: Pamela Hetherington

Immunology and Allergy Clinics of North America (ISSN 0889–8561) is published quarterly by Elsevier Inc., 360 Park Avenue South, New York, NY 10010-1710. Months of issue are February, May, August, and November. Periodicals postage paid at New York, NY and additional mailing offices. Subscription prices are $294.00 per year for US individuals, $417.00 per year for US institutions, $139.00 per year for US students and residents, $361.00 per year for Canadian individuals, $202.00 per year for Canadian students, $518.00 per year for Canadian institutions, $409.00 per year for international individuals, $518.00 per year for international institutions, $202.00 per year for international students. To receive student/resident rate, orders must be accompanied by name of affiliated institution, date of term, and the *signature* of program/residency coordinator on institution letterhead. Orders will be billed at individual rate until proof of status is received. Foreign air speed delivery is included in all *Clinics* subscription prices. All prices are subject to change without notice. **POSTMASTER:** Send address changes to *Immunology and Allergy Clinics of North America,* Elsevier Health Sciences Division, Subscription Customer Service, 3251 Riverport Lane, Maryland Heights, MO 63043. **Customer Service: 1-800-654-2452 (U.S. and Canada); 314-447-8871 (outside U.S. and Canada). Fax: 314-447-8029. E-mail: journalscustomerservice-usa@elsevier.com (for print support); journalsonlinesupport-usa@elsevier.com (for online support).**

Reprints. For copies of 100 or more, of articles in this publication, please contact the Commercial Reprints Department, Elsevier Inc., 360 Park Avenue South, New York, New York 10010-1710. Tel. (212) 633-3812, Fax: (212) 462-1935, E-mail: reprints@elsevier.com.

Immunology and Allergy Clinics of North America is covered in MEDLINE/PubMed (Index Medicus), Current Contents/Life Sciences, Science Citation Index, ISI/BIOMED, Chemical Abstracts, and EMBASE/Excerpta Medica.

Printed and bound by CPI Group (UK) Ltd, Croydon, CR0 4YY

Transferred to Digital Print 2012

Contributors

CONSULTING EDITOR

RAFEUL ALAM, MD, PhD
Veda and Chauncey Ritter Chair in Immunology, Professor and Director, Division of Immunology and Allergy, National Jewish Health; and University of Colorado Health Sciences Center, Denver, Colorado

GUEST EDITOR

ROHIT K. KATIAL, MD, FAAAAI, FACP
Program Director, Adult Allergy and Immunology, Professor of Medicine, Department of Medicine, National Jewish Health, University of Colorado, Denver, Colorado

AUTHORS

RONINA A. COVAR, MD
Associate Professor of Pediatrics, Department of Pediatrics, National Jewish Health, Denver, Colorado

MICHAEL D. DAVIS, BS, RRT
Project Director, Department of Adult Health and Nursing Systems, School of Nursing, Virginia Commonwealth University, Richmond, Virginia

JOHN HUNT, MD
Associate Professor of Pediatrics, Pulmonology, Allergy and Immunology, University of Virginia, Charlottesville, Virginia

ROHIT K. KATIAL, MD, FAAAAI, FACP
Program Director, Adult Allergy and Immunology, Professor of Medicine, Department of Medicine, National Jewish Health, University of Colorado, Denver, Colorado

ALISON MONTPETIT, RN, PhD
Assistant Professor, Department of Adult Health and Nursing Systems, School of Nursing, Virginia Commonwealth University, Richmond, Virginia

NATHAN RABINOVITCH, MD, MPH
Associate Professor, Department of Pediatrics, National Jewish Health, Denver, Colorado

JOSEPH D. SPAHN, MD
Associate Professor of Pediatrics, Ira J. and Jacqueline Neimark Laboratory of Clinical Pharmacology in Pediatrics; Divisions of Pediatric Clinical Pharmacology and Allergy-Clinical Immunology, Department of Pediatrics, National Jewish Health; Department of Pediatrics, University of Colorado Health Sciences Center, Denver, Colorado

LORA STEWART, MD
Allergy & Asthma Care and Prevention Center, Lone Tree, Coloradoz

SALLY E. WENZEL, MD
Professor of Medicine, Director, University of Pittsburgh Asthma Institute at University of Pittsburgh Medical Center, University of Pittsburgh School of Medicine, Pittsburgh, Pennsylvania

Contents

Preface　　ix

Rohit K. Katial

Foreword: Biomarkers in Asthma and Allergy　　xi

Rafeul Alam

Exhaled Nitric Oxide　　347

Lora Stewart and Rohit K. Katial

Nitric oxide (NO) is now considered an important biomarker for respiratory disease. Studies have confirmed that the fractional concentration of exhaled nitric oxide (FENO) is elevated in the airways of patients who have asthma in comparison with controls. The level of FENO correlates well with the presence and level of inflammation, and decreases with glucocorticoid treatment. NO has potential to be used not only as a diagnostic aid but also as a management tool for assessing severity, monitoring response to therapy, and gaining control of asthma symptoms. This article reviews the biology of NO and its role in respiratory disease.

Exhaled Breath Condensate: An Overview　　363

Michael D. Davis, Alison Montpetit, and John Hunt

Exhaled breath condensate (EBC) is a promising source of biomarkers of lung disease. EBC may be thought of either as a body fluid or as a condensate of exhaled gas. There are 3 principal contributors to EBC: variable-sized particles or droplets that are aerosolized from the airway lining fluid, distilled water that condenses from gas phase out of the nearly water-saturated exhalate, and water-soluble volatiles that are exhaled and absorbed into the condensing breath. The nonvolatile constituents and the water-soluble volatile constituents are of particular interest. Several key issues are discussed in this article.

Exhaled Breath Condensate pH Assays　　377

Michael D. Davis and John Hunt

Airway pH is central to the physiologic function and cellular biology of the airway. The causes of airway acidification include (1) hypopharyngeal gastric acid reflux with or without aspiration through the vocal cords, (2) inhalation of acid fog or gas (such as chlorine), and (3) intrinsic airway acidification caused by altered airway pH homeostasis in infectious and inflammatory disease processes. The recognition that relevant airway pH deviations occur in lung diseases is opening doors to new simple and inexpensive therapies. This recognition has resulted partly from the ability to use exhaled breath condensate as a window on airway acid-base balance.

Asthma Biomarkers in Sputum   387

Joseph D. Spahn

> Studies have shown that induced sputum can provide information regarding the cellular and molecular processes involved in asthma and other obstructive pulmonary diseases, and can aid in the diagnosis of asthma and in distinguishing asthma from chronic obstructive pulmonary disease in patients who present with evidence for fixed airflow obstruction. Sputum eosinophils are associated with both asthma severity and level of asthma control. By effectively treating sputum eosinophilia, the number of asthma exacerbations can be significantly reduced compared with managing asthma based on symptoms and lung function.

Tissue-Based and Bronchoalveolar Lavage–Based Biomarkers in Asthma   401

Sally E. Wenzel

> In this article, tissue and bronchoalveolar lavage biomarkers of asthma are evaluated for their use in asthma and evaluated in the context of the phenotype that they may best represent. It is hoped that studies that better link biomarkers to specific phenotypes will eventually improve the ability to evaluate genetic features, diagnose, measure progression, and tailor treatments. Although some biomarkers may only be associated with disease, it is also likely that some may be mechanistically involved. Some of these biomarkers may then also become targets for specific treatment.

Bronchoprovocation Testing in Asthma   413

Rohit K. Katial and Ronina A. Covar

> This article covers the relationships between BHR and airway inflammation. Recent evidence suggests that various commonly used bronchoprovocation challenges (BPCs) differ in their potential to serve as inflammatory biomarkers. The response to direct stimuli depends on the smooth muscle's response to the chemical, whereas in indirect challenges, the reaction is caused by the smooth muscle's responsiveness to the mediators induced by the stimuli. The information obtained from studies with BPC has provided insights into the pathogenesis and pathophysiology of asthma, and the relationships between airway inflammation and bronchial hyper-responsiveness.

Urinary leukotriene E_4 as a Biomarker of Exposure, Susceptibility and Risk in Asthma   433

Nathan Rabinovitch

> Measurement of urinary leukotriene E_4 (uLTE_4) is a sensitive and noninvasive method of assaying total body cysteinyl leukotriene production and changes in cysteinyl leukotriene production. Recent studies have reported on novel uLTE_4 receptor interactions, and new applications for uLTE_4, as a biomarker of environmental exposure to tobacco smoke and ambient air pollution, a predictor of risk for asthma exacerbations related to tobacco smoke, and a marker of susceptibility to leukotriene receptor antagonists.

Index   447

IMMUNOLOGY AND ALLERGY CLINICS OF NORTH AMERICA

FORTHCOMING ISSUES

November 2012
Interstitial Lung Disease
Kevin K. Brown, MD, Aryeh Fischer, MD,
and Jeffrey J. Swigris, DO, MS,
Guest Editors

February 2013
Conditions Mimicking Asthma
Eugene Choo, *Guest Editor*

May 2013
Aspirin and NSAID-Induced Respiratory Diseases
Donald Stevenson, MD,
and Marek Kowalski, MD, *Guest Editors*

RELATED INTEREST

Otolaryngologic Clinics of North America (Volume 45, Issue 4, August 2012)
Pediatric Otolaryngology: Challenges in Multi-system Disease
Austin Rose, MD, *Guest Editor*

NOW AVAILABLE FOR YOUR iPhone and iPad

Preface

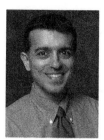

Rohit K. Katial, MD, FAAAAI, FACP
Guest Editor

In 2007, the first issue on Biomarkers in Allergy and Asthma was published. Since then, much has been published on asthma phenotypes and endotypes in an attempt to define various clusters of asthmatics with similar features. Although a variety of parameters have been incorporated into defining these phenotypes, there still continues to be a great need for biomarkers in asthma to objectively define differing disease types within the asthma syndrome. Well-defined biomarkers would ultimately be useful in defining responder profiles to new emerging therapeutics as well as more accurate diagnosis. However, asthma diagnosis and management is still based on clinical symptoms and lung function. This approach, although sound, has significant limitations, including the lack of objective criteria to directly assess airway inflammation, symptom control, and prediction of therapeutic response. In addition, this approach lacks the ability to characterize individual patient differences of a heterogenous disease when relying solely on clinical criteria and lung function.

Due to significant research directly targeted at biomarker development and clinical trials with new biologics using biomarkers such as exhaled nitric oxide, sputum and tissue eosinophilia as endpoints, we decided to issue an update to the 2007 edition. In addition, there has been the approval in the United States of dry powder mannitol for bronchial provocation testing. Such changes were the impetus for this issue, which provides a comprehensive review of the current state of these various biomarkers and their role in the asthma diagnostic and therapeutic algorithm.

Rohit K. Katial, MD, FAAAAI, FACP
Professor of Medicine
Division of Adult Allergy and Immunology
National Jewish Health 1400 Jackson Street
Denver, CO 80206, USA

E-mail address:
KatialR@njhealth.org

Immunol Allergy Clin N Am 32 (2012) ix
http://dx.doi.org/10.1016/j.iac.2012.06.001
0889-8561/12/$ – see front matter © 2012 Elsevier Inc. All rights reserved.

Foreword

Biomarkers in Asthma and Allergy

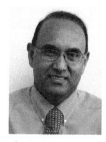

Rafeul Alam, MD, PhD
Consulting Editor

Biomarkers are footprints of disease-related biological processes that are easy to detect and useful in diagnosing and treating the disease condition. Asthma is a heterogeneous disease. For this reason identification of biomarkers that would help diagnose and treat various subtypes of asthma is very important. With the rapid progress in biotechnology, especially the introduction of high throughput and ultrasensitive detection methods, hope has been high that we will soon identify an array of biomarkers that will be useful in clinical practice. There has been steady progress in basic science research and in the identification of promising lead molecules. Some of these molecules have shown promise in discriminating asthmatic patients in their response to various therapeutic agents. A biomarker-based approach allowed resurrection of the anti-IL5 antibody in demonstrating its usefulness in eosinophil-high severe asthmatic patients.[1] Similarly, periostin has been found to identify an asthmatic subtype that is responsive to anti-IL13 intervention.[2] The usefulness of eosinophils (blood and sputum) has been validated in many studies. The usefulness of periostin needs to be validated in broader and more rigorous studies. Nonetheless, these are two good examples of the use of biomarkers in defining asthma subtypes and in predicting their response to therapeutic agents.

Validation of biomarkers has been the biggest challenge as it requires large study samples, ideally involving multiple centers. This lack of validation has been reflected in the recommendation by a recently convened NIH workshop group. The group analyzed existing data and recommended only the following biomarkers for consideration in clinical studies—serologic multi-allergen screen for IgE, total IgE, blood and sputum eosinophils, urinary LTE4, and FENO.[3]

Because of the continued interest in biomarkers and the potential for their use in clinical practice, we felt it was time to revisit the status of biomarker research in asthma

---

Supported by NIH grants RO1 AI091614, PPG HL 36577, and N01 HHSN272200700048C.

Immunol Allergy Clin N Am 32 (2012) xi–xii
http://dx.doi.org/10.1016/j.iac.2012.06.013
0889-8561/12/$ – see front matter © 2012 Elsevier Inc. All rights reserved.

and allergy. We have invited a group of outstanding experts in the field led by Dr Rohit Katial to update us on biomarker research.

Rafeul Alam, MD, PhD
Division of Allergy and Immunology
National Jewish Health and University of Colorado Denver
Health Sciences Center
1400 Jackson Street
Denver, CO 80206, USA

E-mail address:
alamr@njhealth.org

REFERENCES

1. Haldar P, Brightling CE, Hargadon B, et al. Mepolizumab and exacerbations of refractory eosinophilic asthma. N Engl J Med 2009;360:973–84 [Erratum in N Engl J Med 2011;364:588].
2. Corren J, Lemanske RF, Hanania NA, et al. Lebrikizumab treatment in adults with asthma. N Engl J Med 2011;365:1088–98.
3. Szefler SJ, Wenzel S, Brown R, et al. Asthma outcomes: biomarkers. J Allergy Clin Immunol 2012;129(Suppl 3):S9–23.

Exhaled Nitric Oxide

Lora Stewart, MD[a], Rohit K. Katial, MD[b],*

KEYWORDS

- Nitric oxide • Fractional concentration of exhaled NO • Asthma • Glucocorticoids

KEY POINTS

- Continued understanding and correlations of fractional concentration of exhaled nitric oxide (FENO) measurements will likely continue to complement conventional diagnostic and assessment tools for inflammatory lung disease.
- Routine monitoring of FENO and airway eosinophilia may help characterize various asthma phenotypes within the asthma syndrome and guide the appropriate use of inhaled corticosteroids.
- High FENO values (>50 ppb) suggest poor control, the presence of persistent inflammation, and a need for increased anti-inflammatory treatment.
- Low values (<25 ppb) suggest low levels of inflammation and may allow for withdrawal of anti-inflammatory treatment.

Although originally described as endothelial-derived relaxing factor (EDRF), important in arterial tone, nitric oxide (NO) is now considered an important biomarker for respiratory disease.[1,2] Subsequent studies have confirmed that the fractional concentration of exhaled nitric oxide (FENO) is elevated in the airways of patients who have asthma in comparison with controls.[3–6] In addition, the level of FENO correlates well with the presence and level of inflammation, and decreases with glucocorticoid treatment.[6–8] Because the biomarker is noninvasively and easily collected, it has the potential to be used not only as a diagnostic aid but also as a management tool for assessing severity, monitoring response to therapy, and gaining control of asthma symptoms. More recently, the American Thoracic Society has published a clinical guide for application and use of FENO for the clinician.[9] This article reviews the biology of NO and its role in respiratory disease.

BIOLOGY OF NITRIC OXIDE

NO, a gaseous molecule initially believed to be a deleterious component in environmental fumes, became the molecule of the year in 1992 and was found to be an

[a] Allergy & Asthma Care and Prevention Center, 10099 RidgeGate Parkway Suite #400, Lone Tree, CO 80204, USA; [b] National Jewish Health, Division of Allergy and Immunology, 1400 Jackson Street, Denver, CO 80206, USA
* Corresponding author.
E-mail address: KatialR@njhealth.org

Immunol Allergy Clin N Am 32 (2012) 347–362
http://dx.doi.org/10.1016/j.iac.2012.06.005
0889-8561/12/$ – see front matter © 2012 Elsevier Inc. All rights reserved.

important signaling molecule in various biological functions. This gas is abundant in the cardiovascular and respiratory systems, and was initially researched in coronary arteries and termed EDRF. Subsequently, 2 groups in the late 1980s showed that EDRF was the same substance as NO.[1,10]

NO is a free radical gas that diffuses freely from its site of production and is not stored locally. NO has an odd number of electrons and reacts avidly with other molecules, such as oxygen, superoxide, and transition metals.[11] Quickly inactivated by oxygen through conversion to nitrates and nitrites, it also reacts with superoxide anion to yield the unstable product peroxynitrite anion.[11] The latter is a potent oxidant that can nitrosate proteins and lead to lipid-peroxidation products, such as lipoxins. In addition, it is a ubiquitous messenger molecule that in low concentrations may serve as a signaling moiety for regulation of blood flow, nonadrenergic/noncholinergic (NANC) neurotransmission, or platelet activity, and at higher concentrations can exert a cytotoxic effect against tumors or pathogens.[12] NO has been measured in exhaled air in animals and humans and has been shown to correlate with airway inflammation in diseases such as asthma.[13]

NO and related compounds are generated from various resident and inflammatory cells in the human airway.[14] Oxidation of L-arginine in the presence of a set of 3 enzymes known as nitric oxide synthase (NOS) yields NO and L-citrulline.[15,16] This process is both oxygen dependent and NADPH (nicotinamide adenine dinucleotide phosphate) dependent. NOSs are expressed in 3 isoforms that were originally referred to as either constitutive or inducible forms of NOS. The constitutive were classified according to their site of expression: neuronally (nNOS) or endothelial (eNOS). However, these enzymes are now known to be expressed by a wide variety of pulmonary cells and are referred to as NOS1 and NOS3, respectively. The inducible form (iNOS or NOS2) is upregulated by proinflammatory cytokines and stimuli, and is likely expressed continuously by human airway epithelial cells under normal conditions.[17,18]

cNOS is a calcium/calmodulin-dependent enzyme that is activated by increases in intracellular Ca^{2+} and releases NO in picomolar concentrations within seconds of activation. Selective agonists, such as acetylcholine, bradykinin, shear stress, and histamine, can result in increased intracellular Ca^{2+}, thereby activating cNOS.[19] In the lung, NOS1 is expressed in the NANC fibers and generates NO, which acts as a relaxer of smooth muscle.[20,21] NOS3 has been found in pulmonary endothelium as well as bronchial and alveolar epithelium.[22,23] In the bronchial epithelium, NOS3 is believed to function primarily through regulating ciliary beat frequency.[24–26] Both NOS1 and NOS3 are corticosteroid resistant, therefore basal release of NO is not affected by these drugs.[27,28]

iNOS is a calcium/calmodulin-independent enzyme that is induced by tumor necrosis factor α, interferon-γ, interleukin (IL)-1b, viruses, bacteria, allergens, and environmental pollutants. In the respiratory tract, NOS2 has been reported to be expressed in epithelial cells, endothelium, airway and vascular smooth muscle, fibroblasts, mast cells, and neutrophils.[15] In contrast to cNOS, iNOS is glucocorticoid-sensitive and, although some constitutive expression occurs in the airway epithelium, the level of pulmonary expression can be modulated. Once iNOS is induced, the production of NO increases within several hours to nanomolar concentrations, levels that are significantly higher than basal levels resulting from cNOS NO production. In addition to activation from proinflammatory stimuli, other proteins, including kallikrein, Rho-like guanosine triphosphatases, and actinin-4, also regulate NOS2 function.

NOS expression and regulation are just one aspect of the complexities governing the biological activity of NO, and NO itself contributes to several downstream metabolic pathways. NO participates in 3 distinct signaling pathways: (1) heme proteins, (2) S-nitrosylation, and (3) reactivity with products of NADPH oxidase leading to reactive nitrogen species.[29] NO has a particular affinity for the ferrous (Fe^{2+}) moiety of hemoglobin, myoglobin, cytochrome c, and soluble guanylate cyclase (sGC), forming nitrosyl products.[19] Once produced, NO does not have a receptor with which it interacts, and thus freely diffuses, entering cells such as smooth muscle. Once inside cells, it activates soluble guanylyl cyclase (sGC) and converts guanosine triphosphate to cyclic guanosine monophosphate (cGMP), which subsequently exerts downstream effects on protein kinases (cGMP-dependent protein kinases).[19] Nitrosylation is an sGC-independent mechanism of NO activity that results in modification of cysteine residues in target enzymes, such as the production of nitrosothiols. Conversely, the breakdown products of the nitrosothiols serve as NO donors. Therefore, S-nitrosothiols serve as a stable pool of bioactive NO that is resistant to oxidant stress, and offers a mechanism through which to buffer the steady-state flux of NO in biological systems. More importantly, this represents a unique mechanism of cell signaling through posttranslational modification of protein thiol targets.[15,29] NO reaction with superoxide ($O_2.^-$) to form peroxynitrite ($ONOO^-$), a potent oxidant, represents the reactive nitrogen species, the third mechanism of signaling.

The role of NO in the lung includes neurotransmission, vasodilation, bronchial dilatation, and immune enhancement. However, NO has a paradoxic role in a disease such as asthma. For instance, in low concentrations, animal data support the bronchodilatory nature of NO and the NANC-induced bronchodilation effect. However, at higher concentrations, NO seems to act as an inflammatory agent. Elevated exhaled NO values seen in disease states are suspected to be a result of overactivity of oxidative pathways, yielding proinflammatory cytokines and subsequent induction of NOS2 activity. The properties displayed by NO gas have allowed it to be measured in exhaled breath and to serve as a diagnostic and management tool for pulmonary disease.

MEASUREMENT AND INTERPRETATION

Measurement of FENO can be performed with both online or offline techniques, although measurements are more commonly performed online with real-time analyzers. FENO levels are inversely proportional to the expiratory flow rate or flow dependence. High flow rates result in low FENO and, conversely, low flow rates yield higher FENO levels. Flow dependence is partially explained by the fact that FENO is partially derived from a diffusion-based process in the airways.[30,31] Because of this flow dependence, the American Thoracic Society (ATS) and the European Respiratory Society (ERS) adopted a standard for FENO measurements at 50 mL/s. In addition, exhalation against positive pressure causes the velum to close, which excludes upper respiratory NO from falsely raising the measurement of FENO.[30] Online measurements are obtained with a single-breath technique whereby a subject inhales NO free gas to total lung capacity and exhales at 50 mL/s (regulated through an inline resistance and the subject receiving feedback through a computer graphic interface) for approximately 6 seconds, the time required for the FENO levels to plateau. The maneuver is repeated 3 times to assure reproducibility. Further information on this technique is available in the ATS/ERS summary document.[32]

AIRFLOW MODELING

Although asthma involves the large airways and the distal lung, directly assessing the level of small-airway inflammation has been difficult. FENO is believed to provide insight into distal airway inflammation through a noninvasive route. Several investigators have described the sophisticated mathematical modeling, known as the 2-compartment model (alveolar and airway), allowing one to separately derive the relative contribution of the alveolar compartment to the overall NO production.[31–34] This model allows derivation of flow-independent parameters, such as airway-wall NO concentration, airway diffusion factor, and alveolar NO concentration that collectively determine the total exhaled NO production. The relationship between NO output and expiratory flow rate is used to derive the alveolar component. Applying this model to FENO measurements at multiple flow rates has helped to determine the alveolar and airway contributions. At fast flow rates (>50 mL/s) the alveolar contribution to the total NO value predominates, but at slower flow rates (<50 mL/s) airway diffusion predominates.[34]

Paraskakis and colleagues[35] measured FENO at multiple exhalation flow rates in 132 children and confirmed the presence of a small-airway inflammatory process through determining the alveolar NO using the 2-compartment model. In adult asthmatics, Lehtimaki and colleagues[36] measured bronchial flux and alveolar NO, showing a correlation among bronchial hyperresponsiveness, serum eosinophil protein, and bronchial NO, whereas alveolar NO correlated with pulmonary diffusing capacity. This model will likely help define the role of small-airway inflammation in asthma as the relationship between alveolar and bronchial NO and conventional asthma-testing options are better delineated.

NORMAL VALUES

There is ongoing variability between studies attempting to identify a normal reference range within adult and pediatric patient groups. In 2006, Olivieri and colleagues[37] measured levels in more than 200 nonsmoking adults. The levels were collected online with a single-breath technique at 50 mL/s, with a range of 2.6 to 28.8 parts per billion (ppb) found in men and 1.6 to 21.5 ppb in women. The difference between the groups suggested a need to have gender-specific normal values. Olin and colleagues[38] reported a median value of 15.8 ppb with an interquartile range of 11.9 to 21.4 ppb in 179 nonatopic healthy subjects. Buchvald and colleagues[39] studied children aged 4 to 17 years, and measured FENO in more than 400 patients who had a mean value of 9.7 ppb. The upper end of the 95% confidence interval was age dependent, with a value of 15.7 ppb at age 4 years and 25.2 ppb for adolescents.[39] Unfortunately, asthmatic normal values are limited. In the report by Olin and colleagues,[38] the atopic asthmatic cohort showed a median value of 29.8 ppb with an interquartile range of 18.2 to 47.8 ppb.

Olin and colleagues[40] also published FENO values from a random general population sample and found the median value to be 16 ppb, with the 25th to 75th percentiles being 11 and 22.3 ppb, respectively. Height, age, atopy, report of asthma symptoms in the past month, and reported use of inhaled steroids were positively associated with FENO, whereas current smokers had lower values of FENO and gender was not associated with FENO.[40] Another study in pediatric patients demonstrated that race was an important factor as well as age and height in determining baseline FENO values.[41] Rather than using reference values, the current recommendation for interpreting FENO is to use clinical cut points, although well-established cut points are not well validated.[9] The current recommendation is that values less than 25 ppb (or <20 ppb for pediatrics) indicate a lack of eosinophilic inflammation, whereas values greater than 50 ppb (or 35 ppb for pediatrics) are likely to be consistent with eosinophilic inflammation and responsive to corticosteroid treatment. Values between 25 and 50 ppb should be interpreted within the clinical context of each individual patient.[9] Furthermore, based on the authors' unpublished data in asthmatics with ongoing inflammation, even in the presence of oral corticosteroids the FENO levels did not reach the values of controls. These findings suggest that each individual patient who has asthma may have a personal baseline value during periods of excellent control, and this baseline may be used over time to compare future measurements, similar to using values for peak expiratory flow rate (PEFR) or forced expiratory volume in 1 second (FEV_1).

FACTORS AFFECTING NITRIC OXIDE
Eosinophilic Inflammation

Eosinophilic inflammation is a central hallmark of asthma. FENO may be useful in assessing ongoing eosinophilic airway inflammation regardless of degree of symptoms or abnormalities in lung function. Studies confirm a good correlation between FENO and eosinophilia in induced sputum,[42,43] bronchoalveolar lavage (BAL),[44] and tissue.[45–47] Payne and colleagues[46] obtained endobronchial biopsies in asthmatic children aged 6 to 17 years treated with prednisolone. Those who had persistent symptoms and a raised eosinophil score showed higher FENO levels.[29,46] Similarly, in a study of 29 children who had asthma in comparison with controls, Warke and colleagues[44] showed that FENO was positively correlated with BAL eosinophil levels. van den Toorn and colleagues[47] studied adults with asthma who had active disease or were experiencing remission. FENO correlated with major basic protein density in bronchial epithelium. Despite clinical remission, the subjects showed increased FENO, bronchial hyperresponsiveness, and tissue-based eosinophilia, suggesting persistent inflammation despite the lack of clinical symptoms.

The principal author (R.K.) studied FENO levels in patients who had asthma with and without eosinophilic inflammation as measured with induced sputum and endobronchial biopsy. Regardless of oral corticosteroid use, elevated FENO was found in those who had persistent airway eosinophilia when compared with those who did not. The use of oral corticosteroids did not normalize the FENO to levels considered normal (R. Katial, 2006). The occult airway inflammation detected through increased FENO may suggest ongoing airway remodeling despite lack of lung function abnormalities or symptoms. In the future, therapy may be warranted for individuals who have silent but persistent inflammation. Asthma heterogeneity is highlighted by descriptions of variable disease control, presenting symptoms, and types of inflammation. As these data continue to emerge, asthma may be considered a syndrome with differing phenotypes rather than a single disease. This concept of phenotyping asthmatics using FENO was described by Silkoff and colleagues,[13] who showed that elevated FENO measurements identified a subgroup of patients who had severe steroid-refractory asthma and persistent eosinophilia compared with patients who had eosinophilic-negative mild to severe asthma. These data collectively form the basis on which FENO measurements are considered a reliable noninvasive marker for eosinophilic airway inflammation.

Glucocorticoids

In 2003, the US Food and Drug Administration approved the Aerocrine (Stockholm, Sweden) FENO monitoring system (NIOX) for clinical application in patients who have asthma. The labeling of this device was restricted to monitoring the response to anti-inflammatory medications, as an adjunct to established clinical and laboratory assessments, in adults up to 65 years of age and children older than 4 years. FENO as a direct measure of inflammation may be used to determine the response to glucocorticoids. Little and colleagues[48] studied the use of FENO as a marker for response to oral glucocorticoids in 37 adults who had stable asthma, and found that the clinical benefit of oral steroids was greatest in those showing elevated baseline FENO levels. Smith and colleagues[49] showed that FENO measurements were useful in adult patients to determine the benefits of inhaled corticosteroids (ICS) when they studied 52 steroid-naïve subjects who had chronic respiratory symptoms and underwent 4 weeks of treatment with fluticasone. The response to ICS was greatest in the one-third of subjects whose FENO was greater than 47 ppb. In the absence of a high FENO, the response to steroids was less likely, as assessed through symptoms and improvements in spirometry.[49] Similarly, Szefler and colleagues[50] showed that children who had high FENO values were more likely to respond to ICS than those who had lower FENO.

Although these studies show that elevated FENO levels predict steroid responsiveness, the question remains as to whether FENO levels can be used to adjust ICS dose. Two randomized controlled trials used FENO measurements to guide treatment with ICS. The first by Smith and colleagues[49] examined exacerbations and ICS use. In this study, 94 subjects experienced a 40% reduction of ICS dose using a 35 ppb cutoff without any significant difference in the rate of asthma exacerbations. The second study by Pijnenburg and colleagues[51] evaluated 85 children who had asthma. Using a cutoff point of 30 ppb, no significant difference was seen in the cumulative ICS dose between FENO and control groups, but a significant reduction in bronchial hyperresponsiveness was seen in the FENO group, with a concomitant reduction in exacerbations requiring oral steroid use. The differences between the studies may lie in study design. Katsara and colleagues[52] assessed compliance using FENO and a data logger attached to a pressurized meter dose inhaler. This study showed a tendency toward increased FENO with poor compliance. Although these studies do not conclusively prove cause and effect, they suggest the usefulness of FENO as a noninvasive marker in the clinical setting to modulate ICS dose and improve, or at least monitor, patient compliance.

Respiratory Infections

Exhaled NO is increased in association with some viral infections, but not with bacterial infections.[53,54] Infections with rhinovirus results primarily in increased NO formation in the airway, but infection with respiratory syncytial virus and influenza virus appear to result in a reduction in NO formation. The difference is linked to the ability of the virus to induce iNOS expression, although the pathway of this induction is unclear but may be linked to activation of STAT1 via interferons. Bacterial infections, on the other hand, are associated with decreased NO production in the airways.[55]

Other Factors

Other factors may affect FENO levels, including age, gender, and smoking. The effect of age on FENO is limited to children and increases with age until adulthood, then stabilizes.[56,57] In addition, FENO levels seem to be higher in men than women,[40,58] although some reports conflict. Both short-term and chronic smoking cause decreased FENO levels, but these levels are usually still elevated in smoking patients who have asthma.[5,40,59,60]

CLINICAL USE
Asthma

Establishing the diagnosis of asthma is the first step in its clinical management, but is often challenging because no single test is available to diagnose asthma. The National

Asthma Education Prevention Program guidelines define asthma as having 3 components: (1) reversible airflow obstruction, (2) bronchial hyperresponsiveness, and (3) airway inflammation. At present, diagnosis is made from a clinical picture of symptoms plus lung function, which is presumed to be a surrogate marker of underlying airway inflammation. However, these measurements, including FEV_1 and PEFR, can be effort dependent and more realistically represent airway physiology rather than the presence or absence of airway inflammation.[61] In addition, lung-function measurements have the potential risk of missing the presence of mild disease when a patient lacks significant airflow obstruction at the visit.

Because FENO has been positively correlated with the presence of airway eosinophilia and inflammation in some studies, it may be used as a diagnostic test for asthma that truly reflects underlying inflammation. Dupont and colleagues[62] studied 240 steroid-naïve subjects, of whom 160 had asthma based on reversibility in FEV_1 after the administration of a short-acting bronchodilator. In this study, FENO levels were found to have a sensitivity and specificity of 85% and 90%, respectively. Smith and colleagues[63] compared conventional diagnostic tests for asthma with FENO and induced sputum markers. The investigators used bronchial hyperreactivity or β-agonist reversibility as the gold standard for diagnosing asthma and evaluated 47 subjects who had symptoms suggesting asthma, with 17 ultimately diagnosed using their definition. In these individuals, FENO had a sensitivity and specificity of 88% and 79%, respectively; however, the traditional diagnostics, such as FEV_1, PEFR variation more than 20%, changes in FEV_1 and PEFR in response to steroids, and FEV_1/forced vital capacity ratio, all performed poorly compared with both FENO and induced sputum.[63] The combination of FEV_1 and FENO provided an even higher sensitivity (94%) and specificity (93%) for diagnosing asthma.[64]

Although 2 studies[63,65] have shown a poor correlation between FENO and conventional tests, not all patients who have asthma may have an elevated FENO, and thus FENO should be used more appropriately as a complementary test to the current spirometric-based measures. In addition, FENO levels may correlate with eosinophilic inflammation, and in asthmatic patients lacking in eosinophilic inflammation FENO would be normal. The notion that FENO is a surrogate marker for eosinophilic inflammation has been brought into question because of conflicting data. More accurately, exhaled NO is not a marker of atopy per se, but rather a consequence of allergen-induced inflammation and most likely correlates better with tissue eosinophilia rather than with sputum.[66] Because FENO is a noninvasive biomarker, it has excellent potential for assessing and tracking asthma severity, level of asthma control, and responsiveness to inhaled corticosteroid treatment. In one study, asthma control was assessed in 30 patients based on conventional measures of symptoms and lung function. FENO correlated with both asthma control and severity level.[67] To correlate FENO values and asthma control, Jatakanon and colleagues[68] used a steroid reduction model to evaluate 15 patients who had asthma twice weekly over 8 weeks after inhaled steroid reduction. Elevated FENO levels significantly correlated with decreased airway function and FEV_1, and frequency of β-agonist use was also shown to correlate. By contrast, Szefler and colleagues[69] demonstrated that adjusting treatment based on FENO levels in an inner-city asthmatic population resulted in higher doses of ICS compared with management based on symptoms alone. Moreover, there is a small fraction of asthmatic patients in whom FENO fails to improve despite treatment with corticosteroids.[70] In atopic patients with asthma, persistently elevated FENO may be due to ongoing allergen exposure and be related to the level of allergic sensitization.[71] The negative results in the study by Szefler and colleagues[69] may have been due to a combination of ongoing allergen exposure in the inner-city cohort as well as the fact that their asthma and FENO levels were optimized before randomization, leading to difficulty in detecting a difference when using symptoms as an outcome measure. Previous studies showed that monitoring methacholine reactivity as a basis to adjust ICS dose helped reduce asthma exacerbations.[72] A similar study design by Green and colleagues[73] using a treatment strategy based on sputum eosinophilia provided better disease management than a British Thoracic Society guideline algorithm. The subjects in the sputum-based cohort showed significantly lower FENO levels, probably reflecting the reduced eosinophilic inflammation in that group.[73] Finally, when evaluating future risk of asthma, FENO was better than sputum eosinophils at predicting decline in lung function.[74]

Two recent studies evaluated the use of FENO as either an additional diagnostic marker or a treatment criterion in hopes of assessing improved control. The first study by Meyts and colleagues[75] was an office-based evaluation of asthma control in 73 children aged 5 to 18 years. Three levels of control (good, acceptable, and insufficient) were determined based on frequency of β-agonist use, daytime and nighttime symptoms, and spirometry. The subjects determined to have insufficiently controlled disease had the highest median levels of FENO (median 28 ppb), in significant contrast to those who had good and acceptable control.[75] Similar to two other studies,[72,73] a prospective trial by Smith and colleagues[76] evaluated the usefulness of repeat measurements of FENO compared with a guideline-based management strategy. The FENO group experienced a 46% reduction in the number of exacerbations, but based on a predefined cutoff for analysis this reduction did not reach statistical significance. However, a statistically significant reduction occurred in mean ICS use over 12 months in the group managed using FENO measurements.[76] Results of these studies collectively support the concept that using a direct measure of inflammation, such as FENO, may lead to more effective disease management, gauged by minimizing exacerbations and optimizing medication use. A recent study evaluating the efficacy of lebrikizumab (anti–IL-13) for asthma found that patients with higher FENO were associated with better response to treatment.[77] By contrast, mepolizumab (anti–IL-5 monoclonal antibody) treatment had no effect on FENO levels.[78] Although these varied results may seem inconsistent initially, understanding the signaling pathway for FENO sheds light on these results and a better understanding of FENO as a diagnostic marker. Because iNOS is activated by STAT1 and STAT6, IL-4 and IL-13, which upregulate STAT6, would in turn be associated with higher FENO levels. On the other hand, IL-5 upregulates STAT5, which does not have an effect on iNOS or FENO levels. Understanding this pathway further supports the idea that FENO is not a surrogate marker for sputum eosinophils but rather a parallel marker of airway inflammation. FENO is likely a better marker for local airway mucosal or bronchial inflammation because it correlates well with the IL-4/IL-13/STAT6 pathway, and this is not purely related to eosinophilic counts.

Chronic Obstructive Pulmonary Disease

Because of its usefulness in diagnosing and assessing inflammation in asthma, potential use of FENO measurements for diagnosing chronic obstructive pulmonary disease (COPD) was an obvious next step for this biomarker. Unfortunately, FENO is not elevated in stable COPD and therefore is not a useful diagnostic biomarker.[79,80] In addition, because glucocorticoid therapy has limited value in COPD treatment, the relationship between FENO values and steroid use is not as well correlated. The low levels of FENO for COPD are likely caused by several factors, including the prevalence of cigarette smoking and predominance of neutrophilic inflammation seen in these patients.[80] A small but detectable difference is seen in patients who have COPD and are current smokers, compared with ex-smoking patients or those who never smoked.[81] FENO levels correlate well with eosinophilic inflammation rather than neutrophilic inflammation. FENO may have a role in patients who have unstable COPD and those experiencing COPD exacerbations. These patients were found to have elevated FENO levels when compared with patients who had stable COPD (both smokers and ex-smokers).[82] During acute COPD exacerbations, the level of eosinophilic inflammation increases, which may explain the increase seen in FENO.[83] This increase is smaller than that seen in association with asthma exacerbations, probably because the inflammation present is different, and is without eosinophilic degranulation and lower activation of iNOS.[84]

In the lungs of patients who had COPD, one study showed a correlation between FENO levels and diffusing capacity that did not correlate with glucocorticoid treatment.[85] COPD exacerbations are often characterized by acidosis, which may have a vasodilatory influence on the vasculature, and could lead to increased myeloperoxidase activity in the lung and subsequent increased FENO levels.[86] Therefore, the mild elevation in FENO seen with COPD exacerbations may actually be caused by altered pulmonary function and gas exchange rather than inflammation. The usefulness of FENO measurement and monitoring in COPD patients is currently unclear and requires additional studies to delineate this aspect.

Cystic Fibrosis

FENO measurements in patients who have cystic fibrosis have been reported to be low to normal compared with those of healthy controls.[87–91] In addition, although an older citation reports that FENO did not distinguish between genotype or infection status,[92] a more recent study reported lower FENO levels in patients who had associated pancreatic insufficiency.[90] Throughout all studies evaluating cystic fibrosis and FENO, one consistent finding is that FENO levels in patients who have cystic fibrosis are always lower than comparison patients who have asthma. Although this finding was initially somewhat counterintuitive, because cystic fibrosis is clearly an inflammatory lung condition, the inflammation seen in cystic fibrosis clearly has a neutrophilic predominance compared with the eosinophilic inflammation of asthma and atopy.[93] The low levels of FENO has been hypothesized to have several possible causes, including poor gas diffusion through the thick mucus found in the lungs of patients who have cystic fibrosis, bacterial consumption of NO, and decreased production of NO. Grasemann and colleagues[94] recently compared different NOS1 genotypes in patients who had cystic fibrosis and bacterial colonization, and found that certain alleles were associated with both lower levels of FENO and colonization with *Pseudomonas aeruginosa* and *Aspergillus fumigatus*. The role of FENO in cystic fibrosis still remains to be fully clarified, but has potential to be an adjunct in both diagnosis and management.

Interstitial Lung Disease

Interstitial lung disease (ILD) is a group of lung diseases consisting of several different underlying pathophysiologic states, all of which result in inflammation and subsequent fibrosis of the lungs. The role of FENO in the diagnosis and treatment of ILD continues to expand and gain better understanding. FENO does seem to have a role in patients who have scleroderma, in which FENO levels were found to be increased in patients who had scleroderma and ILD compared with both patients who had scleroderma without ILD and normal controls.[95]

The usefulness of FENO levels has not been found for all forms of ILD. In fact, FENO does not seem to be different in individuals who have pulmonary sarcoidosis in comparison with healthy controls.[96] In addition to having normal FENO levels, no correlation was seen with disease severity as judged with high-resolution computed tomography or lung function. In the future, FENO measurement may serve as a noninvasive surveillance tool for the development and progression of certain subsets of ILD.

Primary Ciliary Dyskinesia

Primary ciliary dyskinesia (PCD) is a congenital disease characterized by abnormal cilia motility. Patients who have PCD have decreased mucociliary clearance, which results in subsequent pulmonary disease, including chronic infection, inflammation, and bronchiectasis. Patients who have this disease also have very low and stable levels of FENO. Subsequently, FENO has been suggested as a diagnostic tool when evaluating patients who have recurrent pulmonary symptoms to distinguish PCD from other bronchiectatic lung diseases, such as cystic fibrosis and asthma.[97,98] However, although FENO may be used as a screening tool, the diagnosis of PCD should be confirmed with biopsy. The very low levels of FENO are especially intriguing, because in many other pulmonary conditions FENO correlates well with the level of inflammation present. In addition, the very low levels of FENO seen in patients who had PCD did not seem to be modified by the presence or lack of atopic status[97] or the use of ICS.[98] The cause of the low FENO values seen in PCD remains to be confirmed, but is hypothesized to be related to the abnormal cilia function that may lead to reduced NOS output and subsequent reduced NO production.[97] Moreover, the inflammation present in PCD is predominantly neutrophilic rather than eosinophilic.[99] Finally, treating patients who have PCD with L-arginine, causing normalization of NO levels, has been shown to result in improved mucociliary transport.[100,101] This finding supports the hypothesis that the lack of airway NO not only is characteristic of the disease but also may play a role in the pathology.

Bronchiolitis Obliterans

Bronchiolitis obliterans syndrome (BOS) is a clinical syndrome of irreversible and progressive lung destruction in patients who have undergone pulmonary transplantation, believed to be caused by chronic rejection. Unfortunately, despite lung transplantation being a well-established treatment option for patients who have end-stage lung disease, nearly 50% of patients develop this complication 3 years or more after receiving their allograft.[102] In addition, early detection and additional immunosuppression in patients who have progressive BOS improves survival, but limited markers exist for detecting progressive BOS.[103] Evidence now shows that FENO levels correlate well with progressive stages of BOS and loss of lung function. Serial measurement of FENO has potential for monitoring patients after transplantation and guiding intervention with additional therapy to better manage and treat BOS.[104]

SUMMARY

Before the use of FENO, direct assessment of airway inflammation was limited to invasive techniques. Continued understanding and correlations of FENO measurements will likely continue to complement conventional diagnostic and assessment tools for inflammatory lung disease. Because the technique is noninvasive, it will probably be used regularly not only for initial diagnosis but also for routine assessment of disease severity, response to treatment, and compliance. Furthermore, routine monitoring of FENO and airway eosinophilia may help characterize various asthma phenotypes within the asthma syndrome and guide the appropriate use of ICS. Although a precise normal is still awaited, good data exist for high positive and negative predictive values for diagnosing and treating asthma at both ends of the spectrum of FENO values. High

FENO values (>50 ppb) suggest poor control, the presence of persistent inflammation, and a need for increased anti-inflammatory treatment. Low values (<25 ppb) suggest low levels of inflammation and may allow for withdrawal of anti-inflammatory treatment. At present, FENO serves as a complementary tool in managing patients who have asthma and other inflammatory diseases in addition to conventional measures of symptom control and response to therapy, while larger studies are awaited to define normative ranges for all patients.

ACKNOWLEDGMENTS

The authors would like to thank Dierdre Versluis for her assistance in the preparation of this article.

REFERENCES

1. Palmer RM, Ferrige AG, Moncada S. Nitric oxide release accounts for the biological activity of endothelium-derived relaxing factor. Nature 1987;327:524–6.
2. Gustafsson LE, Leone AM, Persson MG, et al. Endogenous nitric oxide is present in the exhaled air of rabbits, guinea pigs and humans. Biochem Biophys Res Commun 1991;181:852–7.
3. Alving K, Weitzberg E, Lundberg JM. Increased amount of nitric oxide in exhaled air of asthmatics. Eur Respir J 1993;6:1368–70.
4. Kharitonov SA, Yates D, Robbins RA, et al. Increased nitric oxide in exhaled air of asthmatic patients. Lancet 1994;343:133–5.
5. Persson MG, Zetterstrom O, Agrenius V, et al. Single-breath nitric oxide measurements in asthmatic patients and smokers. Lancet 1994;343:146–7.
6. Yates DH, Kharitonov SA, Robbins RA, et al. Effect of a nitric oxide synthase inhibitor and a glucocorticosteroid on exhaled nitric oxide. Am J Respir Crit Care Med 1995;152:892–6.
7. Kharitonov SA, Yates DH, Barnes PJ. Inhaled glucocorticoids decrease nitric oxide in exhaled air of asthmatic patients. Am J Respir Crit Care Med 1996; 153:454–7.
8. Massaro AF, Gaston B, Kita D, et al. Expired nitric oxide levels during treatment of acute asthma. Am J Respir Crit Care Med 1995;152:800–3.
9. Dweik R, Boggs PB, Erzurum SC, et al. An official ATS clinical practice guideline: interpretation of exhaled nitric oxide levels for clinical applications. Am J Respir Crit Care Med 2011;184:602–15.
10. Ignarro LJ, Buga GM, Wood KS, et al. Endothelium-derived relaxing factor produced and released from artery and vein is nitric oxide. Proc Natl Acad Sci U S A 1987;84:9265–9.
11. Kerwin JF, Heller M. The arginine-nitric oxide pathway: a target for new drugs. Med Res Rev 1994;14:23–74.
12. Moncada S, Higgs A. The L-arginine-nitric oxide pathway. N Engl J Med 1993; 329:2002–12.
13. Silkoff PE, Lent A, Busacker A, et al. Exhaled nitric oxide identifies the persistent eosinophilic phenotype in severe refractory asthma. J Allergy Clin Immunol 2005;116:1249–55.
14. Gaston B, Kobzik L, Stamler JS. Distribution of nitric oxide synthase in the lung. In: Zapol WM, Bloch KD, editors. Nitric oxide and the lung. New York: Dekker; 1997. p. 75–86.
15. Ricciardolo FL, Sterk PJ, Gaston B, et al. Nitric oxide in health and disease of the respiratory system. Physiol Rev 2004;84:731–65.

16. Förstermann U, Schmidt HH, Pollock JS, et al. Isoforms of nitric oxide synthase: characterization and purification from different cell types. Biochem Pharmacol 1991;42:1849–57.

17. Guo FH, De Raeve HR, Rice TW, et al. Continuous nitric oxide synthesis by inducible nitric oxide synthase in normal human airway epithelium in vivo. Proc Natl Acad Sci U S A 1995;92:7809–13.

18. Fischer A, Folkerts G, Geppetti P, et al. Mediators of asthma: nitric oxide. Pulm Pharmacol Ther 2002;15:73–81.

19. Yates DH. Role of exhaled nitric oxide in asthma. Immunol Cell Biol 2001;79: 178–90.

20. Belvisi MG, Stretton CD, Yacoub M, et al. Nitric oxide is the endogenous neurotransmitter of bronchodilator nerves in humans. Eur J Pharmacol 1992;210: 221–2.

21. Li CG, Rand MJ. Evidence that part of the NANC relaxant response of guinea pig trachea to electrical field stimulation is mediated by nitric oxide. Br J Pharmacol 1991;102:91–4.

22. Shaul PW, North AJ, Wu LC, et al. Endothelial nitric oxide synthase is expressed in cultured human bronchiolar epithelium. J Clin Invest 1994;94:2231–6.

23. Pechkovsky DV, Zissel G, Goldmann T, et al. Pattern of NOS2 and NOS3 mRNA expression in human A549 cells and primary cultured AEC II. Am J Physiol Lung Cell Mol Physiol 2002;282:L684–92.

24. Li D, Shirakami G, Zhan X, et al. Regulation of ciliary beat frequency by the nitric oxide cyclic guanosine monophosphate signaling pathway in rat airway epithelial cells. Am J Respir Cell Mol Biol 2000;23:175–81.

25. Getsberg I, Hellman V, Fainshtein M, et al. Intracellular Ca^{2+} regulates the phosphorylation and the dephosphorylation of ciliary proteins via the NO pathway. J Gen Physiol 2004;124:527–40.

26. Jain B, Rubinstein I, Robbins RA, et al. Modulation of airway epithelial cell ciliary beat frequency by nitric oxide. Biochem Biophys Res Commun 1993; 191:83–8.

27. Di Rosa M, Radomski M, Carnuccio R, et al. Glucocorticosteroids inhibit the expression of nitric oxide synthase in macrophages. Biochem Biophys Res Commun 1990;172:1246–52.

28. Radomski MW, Palmer RM, Moncada S. Glucocorticoids inhibit the expression of an inducible, but not the constitutive, nitric oxide synthase in vascular endothelial cells. Proc Natl Acad Sci U S A 1990;87:10043–7.

29. Bove PF, Van der Vliet A. Nitric oxide and reactive nitrogen species in airway epithelial signaling and inflammation. Free Radic Biol Med 2006;41:515–27.

30. Silko PE, McClean PA, Slutsky AS, et al. Marked flow-dependence of exhaled nitric oxide using a new technique to exclude nasal nitric oxide. Am J Respir Crit Care Med 1997;155:260–7.

31. Silko PE, Sylvester JT, Zamel N, et al. Airway nitric oxide diffusion in asthma: role in pulmonary function and bronchial responsiveness. Am J Respir Crit Care Med 2000;161:1218–28.

32. ATS/ERS recommendations for standardized procedures for the online and offline measurement of exhaled lower respiratory nitric oxide and nasal nitric oxide, 2005. Am J Respir Crit Care Med 2005;171:912–30.

33. George SC, Hogman M, Permutt S, et al. Modeling pulmonary nitric oxide exchange. J Appl Physiol 2004;96:831–9.

34. Tsoukias NM, George SC. A two-compartment model of pulmonary nitric oxide exchange dynamics [see comment]. J Appl Physiol 1998;85:653–66.

35. Paraskakis E, Brindicci C, Fleming L, et al. Measurement of bronchial and alve-
    olar nitric oxide production in normal children and children with asthma. Am J
    Respir Crit Care Med 2006;174:260–7.
36. Lehtimaki L, Kankaanranta H, Saarelainen S, et al. Extended exhaled NO
    measurement differentiates between alveolar and bronchial inflammation. Am
    J Respir Crit Care Med 2001;163:1557–61.
37. Olivieri M, Talamini G, Corradi M, et al. Reference values for exhaled nitric oxide
    (REVENO) study. Respir Res 2006;7:94.
38. Olin AC, Alving K, Toren K. Exhaled nitric oxide: relation to sensitization and
    respiratory symptoms. Clin Exp Allergy 2004;34:221–6.
39. Buchvald F, Baraldi E, Carraro S, et al. Measurements of exhaled nitric oxide in
    healthy subjects age 4 to 17 years. J Allergy Clin Immunol 2005;115:1130–6.
40. Olin AC, Rosengren A, Thelle DS, et al. Height, age, and atopy are associated
    with fraction of exhaled nitric oxide in a large adult general population sample.
    Chest 2006;130(5):1319–25.
41. Kovesi T, Kulka R, Dales R. Exhaled nitric oxide concentration is affected by age,
    height and race in healthy 9- to 12-year-old children. Chest 2008;133:169–75.
42. Berlyne GS, Parameswaran K, Kamada D, et al. A comparison of exhaled nitric
    oxide and induced sputum as markers of airway inflammation. J Allergy Clin Im-
    munol 2000;106:638–44.
43. Jatakanon A, Lim S, Kharitonov SA, et al. Correlation between exhaled nitric
    oxide, sputum eosinophils, and methacholine responsiveness in patients with
    mild asthma. Thorax 1998;53:91–5.
44. Warke TJ, Fitch PS, Brown V, et al. Exhaled nitric oxide correlates with airway
    eosinophils in childhood asthma. Thorax 2002;57:383–7.
45. Brightling CE, Symon FA, Birring SS, et al. Comparison of airway immunopa-
    thology of eosinophilic bronchitis and asthma. Thorax 2003;58:528–32.
46. Payne DN, Adcock IM, Wilson NM, et al. Relationship between exhaled nitric
    oxide and mucosal eosinophilic inflammation in children with difficult asthma,
    after treatment with oral prednisolone [see comment]. Am J Respir Crit Care
    Med 2001;164:1376–81.
47. van den Toorn LM, Overbeek SE, de Jongste JC, et al. Airway inflammation is present
    during clinical remission of atopic asthma [published erratum appears in Am J Respir
    Crit Care Med 2002;166:1143]. Am J Respir Crit Care Med 2001;164:2107–13.
48. Little SA, Chalmers GW, MacLeod KJ, et al. Noninvasive markers of airway
    inflammation as predictors of oral steroid responsiveness in asthma. Thorax
    2000;55:232–4.
49. Smith AD, Cowan JO, Brassett KP, et al. Exhaled nitric oxide: a predictor of
    steroid response. Am J Respir Crit Care Med 2005;172:453–9.
50. Szefler SJ, Phillips BR, Martinez FD, et al. Characterization of within-subject
    responses to fluticasone and montelukast in childhood asthma [see comment].
    J Allergy Clin Immunol 2005;115:233–42.
51. Pijnenburg MW, Bakker EM, Hop WC, et al. Titrating steroids on exhaled nitric
    oxide in children with asthma: a randomized controlled trial. Am J Respir Crit
    Care Med 2005;172:831–6.
52. Katsara M, Donnelly D, Iqbal S, et al. Relationship between exhaled nitric oxide
    levels and compliance with inhaled corticosteroids in asthmatic children. Respir
    Med 2006;100:1512–7.
53. Kharitonov SA, Yates D, Barnes PJ. Increased nitric oxide in exhaled air of
    normal human subjects with upper respiratory tract infections. Eur Respir J
    1995;8:295–7.

54. Carraro S, Andreola B, Alinova R, et al. Exhaled leukotriene B4 in children with community acquired pneumonia. Pediatr Pulmonol 2008;43:982–6.
55. Papi A, Bellettato CM, Braccioni F, et al. Infections and airway inflammation in chronic obstructive pulmonary disease severe exacerbations. Am J Respir Crit Care Med 2006;173:1114–21.
56. Franklin PJ, Taplin R, Stick SM. A community study of exhaled nitric oxide in healthy children. Am J Respir Crit Care Med 1999;159:69–73.
57. Kissoon N, Duckworth LJ, Blake KV, et al. Exhaled nitric oxide concentrations: online versus offline values in healthy children. Pediatr Pulmonol 2002;33: 283–92.
58. Tsang KW, Ip SK, Leung R, et al. Exhaled nitric oxide: the effects of age, gender and body size. Lung 2001;179:83–91.
59. Chambers DC, Tunnicliffe WS, Ayres JG. Acute inhalation of cigarette smoke increases lower respiratory tract nitric oxide concentrations. Thorax 1998;53: 677–9.
60. Horvath I, Donnelly LE, Kiss A, et al. Exhaled nitric oxide and hydrogen peroxide concentrations in asthmatic smokers. Respiration 2004;71:463–8.
61. Sont JK, Han J, van Krieken JM, et al. Relationship between the inflammatory infiltrate in bronchial biopsy specimens and clinical severity of asthma in patients treated with inhaled steroids. Thorax 1996;51:496–502.
62. Dupont LJ, Demedts MG, Verleden GM. Prospective evaluation of the validity of exhaled nitric oxide for the diagnosis of asthma. Chest 2003;123:751–6.
63. Smith AD, Cowan JO, Filsell S, et al. Diagnosing asthma: comparisons between exhaled nitric oxide measurements and conventional tests. Am J Respir Crit Care Med 2004;169:473–8.
64. Smith AD, Taylor DR. Is exhaled nitric oxide measurement a useful clinical test in asthma? Curr Opin Allergy Clin Immunol 2005;5:49–56.
65. Zietkowski Z, Bodzenta-Lukaszyk A, Tomasiak MM, et al. Comparison of exhaled nitric oxide measurement with conventional tests in steroid-naive asthma patients. J Investig Allergol Clin Immunol 2006;16:239–46.
66. Alving K, Mailovschi A. Basic aspects of exhaled nitric oxide. Eur Respir Mon 2010;49:1–31.
67. Delgado-Corcoran C, Kissoon N, Murphy SP, et al. Exhaled nitric oxide reflects asthma severity and asthma control. Pediatr Crit Care Med 2004;5:48–52.
68. Jatakanon A, Lim S, Barnes PJ. Changes in sputum eosinophils predict loss of asthma control. Am J Respir Crit Care Med 2000;161:64–72.
69. Szefler S, Mitchell H, Sorkness C, et al. Management of asthma based on exhaled nitric oxide in addition to guideline-based treatment for inner-city adolescents and young adults: a randomized controlled trial. Lancet 2008;372:1065–72.
70. Pijnenburg M, Bakker E, Lever S, et al. High fractional concentration of nitric oxide in exhaled air despite steroid treatment in asthmatic children. Clin Exp Allergy 2005;35:920–5.
71. Buchvald F, Eiberg H, Bisgaard H. Heterogeneity of FeNO response to inhaled steroid in asthmatic children. Clin Exp Allergy 2003;33:1735–40.
72. Sont JK, Willems LN, Bel EH, et al. Clinical control and histopathologic outcome of asthma when using airway hyperresponsiveness as an additional guide to long-term treatment. The AMPUL Study Group. Am J Respir Crit Care Med 1999;159:1043–51.
73. Green RH, Brightling CE, Woltmann G, et al. Analysis of induced sputum in adults with asthma: identification of subgroup with isolated sputum neutrophilia and poor response to inhaled corticosteroids. Thorax 2002;57:875–9.

74. van Veen I, Ten Brinke A, Sterk P, et al. Exhaled nitric oxide predicts lung function decline in difficult-to-treat asthma. Eur Respir J 2008;32:344–9.
75. Meyts I, Proesmans M, De Boeck K. Exhaled nitric oxide corresponds with office evaluation of asthma control. Pediatr Pulmonol 2003;36:283–9.
76. Smith AD, Cowan JO, Brassett KP, et al. Use of exhaled nitric oxide measurements to guide treatment in chronic asthma. N Engl J Med 2005;352:2163–73.
77. Corren J, Lemanske R, Hanania N, et al. Lebrikizumab treatment in adults with asthma. N Engl J Med 2011;365:1088–98.
78. Haldar P, Brightling C, Hargadon B, et al. Mepolizumab and exacerbations of refractory eosinophilic asthma. N Engl J Med 2009;360:973–84.
79. Robbins RA, Floreani AA, Von Essen SG, et al. Measurement of exhaled nitric oxide by three different techniques. Am J Respir Crit Care Med 1996;153: 1631–5.
80. Corradi M, Majori M, Cacciani GC, et al. Increased exhaled nitric oxide in patients with stable chronic obstructive pulmonary disease. Thorax 1999;54: 572–5.
81. Bhowmilk A, Seemungal TA, Donaldson GC, et al. Effects of exacerbations and seasonality on exhaled nitric oxide in COPD. Eur Respir J 2005;26:1009–15.
82. Maziak W, Loukides S, Culpitt S, et al. Exhaled nitric oxide in chronic obstructive pulmonary disease. Am J Respir Crit Care Med 1998;157:998–1002.
83. Rutgers SR, van der Mark TW, Coers W, et al. Markers of nitric oxide metabolism in sputum and exhaled air are not increased in chronic obstructive pulmonary disease. Thorax 1999;54:576–80.
84. Jeffery PK. Structural and inflammatory changes in COPD: a comparison with asthma. Thorax 1998;53:129–36.
85. Ansarin K, Chatkin JM, Ferreira IM, et al. Exhaled nitric oxide in chronic obstructive pulmonary disease: relationship to pulmonary function. Eur Respir J 2001;17:934–8.
86. Pedoto A, Caruso JE, Nandi J, et al. Acidosis stimulates nitric oxide production and lung damage in rats. Am J Respir Crit Care Med 1999;159:397–402.
87. Elphick HE, Demoncheaux EA, Ritson S, et al. Exhaled nitric oxide is reduced in infants with cystic fibrosis. Thorax 2001;56:151–2.
88. Franklin PJ, Hall GL, Moeller A, et al. Exhaled nitric oxide is not reduced in infants with cystic fibrosis. Eur Respir J 2006;27:350–3.
89. Grasemann H, Michler E, Wallot M, et al. Decreased concentration of exhaled nitric oxide (NO) in patients with cystic fibrosis. Pediatr Pulmonol 1997;24:173–7.
90. Keen C, Olin AC, Edenoft A, et al. Airway nitric oxide in patient with cystic fibrosis is associated with pancreatic function, pseudomonas infection, and polyunsaturated fatty acids. Chest 2007;131:1857–64.
91. Lundberg JO, Nordvall SL, Weitzberg E, et al. Exhaled NO in pediatric asthma and cystic fibrosis. Arch Dis Child 1996;75:323–6.
92. Thomas SR, Kharitonov SA, Scott SF, et al. Nasal and exhaled nitric oxide is reduced in adult patients with cystic fibrosis and does not correlate with cystic fibrosis genotype. Chest 2000;117:1085–9.
93. Armstrong DS, Grimwood K, Carlin JB, et al. Lower airway inflammation in infants and young children with cystic fibrosis. Am J Respir Crit Care Med 1997;156:1197–204.
94. Grasemann H, Knauer N, Busher R, et al. Airway nitric oxide levels in cystic fibrosis patients are related to a polymorphism in the neuronal nitric oxide synthase gene. Am J Respir Crit Care Med 2000;162:2172–6.
95. Tiev KP, Cabane J, Aubourg F, et al. Severity of scleroderma lung disease is related to alveolar concentration of nitric oxide. Eur Respir J 2007;30:26–30.

96. Wilsher ML, Fergusson W, Milne D, et al. Exhaled nitric oxide in sarcoidosis. Thorax 2005;60:967–70.
97. Narang I, Ersu R, Wilson NM, et al. Nitric oxide in chronic airway inflammation in children: diagnostic use and pathophysiological significance. Thorax 2002;57: 586–9.
98. Horvath I, Loukides S, Wodehouse T, et al. Comparison of exhaled and nasal nitric oxide and exhaled carbon monoxide levels in bronchiectatic patients with and without primary ciliary dyskinesia. Thorax 2003;58:68–72.
99. Zihlif N, Paraskakis E, Lex C, et al. Correlation between cough frequency and airway inflammation in children with primary ciliary dyskinesia. Pediatr Pulmonol 2005;39:551–7.
100. Loukides S, Kharitonov SA, Wodehouse T, et al. Effect of L-arginine on mucociliary function in primary ciliary dyskinesia. Lancet 1998;352:371–2.
101. Kharitonov SA, Lubec G, Lubec B, et al. L-arginine increases exhaled nitric oxide in normal human subjects. Clin Sci 1995;88:135–9.
102. Sundaresan S, Trulock EP, Mohanakumar T, et al. Prevalence and outcome of bronchiolitis obliterans syndrome after lung transplantation. Washington University Lung Transplant Group. Ann Thorac Surg 1995;60:1341–6.
103. Heng D, Sharples LD, McNeil K, et al. Bronchiolitis obliterans syndrome: incidence, natural history, prognosis and risk factors. J Heart Lung Transplant 1998;17:1255–63.
104. Brugiere O, Thabut G, Mal H, et al. Exhaled NO may predict the decline in lung function in bronchiolitis obliterans syndrome. Eur Respir J 2005;25:813–9.

Exhaled Breath Condensate
An Overview

Michael D. Davis, BS, RRT[a],*, Alison Montpetit, RN, PhD[a],
John Hunt, MD[b]

KEYWORDS

- Exhaled breath condensate • Biomarker • Airway • Exhalate

KEY POINTS

- Exhaled Breath Condensate (EBC) is a promising source of biomarkers of lung disease.
- EBC is composed of three primary constituents: aerosolized particles of airway lining fluid (ALF), distilled water, and water-soluble volatiles.
- EBC can be safely and easily collected from spontaneously breathing subjects and from patients undergoing mechanical ventilation.
- One of the major needs in EBC research is the establishment of methodological standards and normative values specific to each EBC biomarker.

Exhaled breath condensate (EBC) is a promising source of biomarkers of lung disease. EBC is not a biomarker, but a matrix in which biomarkers may be identified, so, in that way, it is equivalent to blood, sweat, tears, urine, and saliva. EBC may be thought of either as a body fluid or as a condensate of exhaled gas (and therefore not a body fluid). This issue is relevant because of potential regulatory issues involved with laboratory assessment of body fluids.

There are 3 principal contributors to EBC.[1] First are variable-sized particles or droplets that are aerosolized from the airway lining fluid (ALF); such particles presumably reflect the fluid itself. Second is distilled water that condenses from gas phase out of the nearly water-saturated exhalate, substantially diluting the aerosolized ALF. Third are water-soluble volatiles that are exhaled and absorbed into the condensing breath. Interest lies both in the nonvolatile constituents, mostly derived from the ALF particles,

Conflict of interest: JH is a cofounder of Respiratory Research, Inc, which manufactures exhaled breath condensate collection equipment. MD and AM are supported by grant K99/R00 NR012016 from the National Institute of Nursing Research.
[a] Department of Adult Health and Nursing Systems, School of Nursing, Virginia Commonwealth University, 1100 East Leigh Street, P.O. Box 980567, Richmond, VA 23298-0567, USA;
[b] Department of Pediatrics, Pulmonology, Allergy & Immunology, University of Virginia, Box 800386, Charlottesville, VA 22908, USA
* Corresponding author.
E-mail address: mdavis35@vcu.edu

Immunol Allergy Clin N Am 32 (2012) 363–375
http://dx.doi.org/10.1016/j.iac.2012.06.014
0889-8561/12/$ – see front matter
immunology.theclinics.com

and in the water-soluble volatile constituents that are found in substantially higher concentrations and are therefore more readily assayed than the nonvolatile compounds.

EBC research has advanced gradually, with the debates surrounding an emerging field helping to pose questions and gradually leading to answers. Several key issues are discussed in this article.

SOURCE OF EBC BIOMARKERS

Little work has been done to understand the nature and source of the exhaled particles/droplets that are part of the EBC matrix. That micrometer and submicrometer droplets emanate from the mouth or endotracheal tube in exhaled breath has been confirmed by laser particle counters,[2,3] and such particles are the only explanation for the presence of nonvolatile constituents in EBC such as cytokines[4] and sodium ions.[5] However, how these particles form and change during exhalation before leaving the body is the subject of speculation. Theories include that small amounts of ALF are torn from the airway surface when turbulence applies energy to the airway wall, similar to spray arising from whitecaps on the ocean on a windy day. Energy to overcome surface tension may also be applied to the wall when closed airways/alveoli pop open during inspiration, potentially creating exhalable particles. Although surfactant and surfactant proteins found in EBC[6] have been suggested to indicate an alveolar origin of the exhaled particles, this is unlikely, for alveolar fluids can move proximally in the airway.

The size of the particles that are measured rapidly exiting the mouth during expiration may be affected by condensation or evaporation. Size and numerical measurements by laser particle counters therefore reflect the particle size entering the counter, not necessarily the particle size initially generated from the airway lining surface.

PARTICLE SIZE

One 10-μm particle entering a sample of EBC can supply 1 million times the quantity of nonvolatiles to a sample of EBC as a 0.1-μm particle. However, there is skewing of the exhaled particle sizes toward the smaller particles.[3] Overall, the relative contribution to EBC of the nonvolatile constituent of the different sized particles remains unknown.

OROPHARYNGEAL CONTRIBUTION TO EBC

In oral EBC collections, there is no reason to suspect that particles cannot be released from the oral and retropharyngeal mucosa into the airstream, with the potential to contaminate what might otherwise be a pure lower airway sample. Furthermore, depending in part on the EBC collection equipment, gross or microscopic salivary contamination of EBC can occur.[7] Some subjects simply drool during collection, affirming the need for salivary trapping systems to be in place. Measures of salivary amylase are often used to test for the presence of salivary contamination. Most investigators find that no amylase is identified in most samples, although those using higher sensitivity assays tend to report the presence of measurable amylase in a subset of samples.[7] The amylase assays are imperfect and, as with other protein assays in EBC, suffer from a potentially substantial amount of false-positivity and false-negativity. Excessive reliance on any protein assay in EBC has often led to errors, and this may be the case for amylase measures as well. Measurable phosphate has also been suggested to be a reliable indicator of salivary contamination.[8] One group concluded that saliva is the source of less than 10% of respiratory droplets.[9]

The ratios among various nonvolatile compounds in EBC have been found to be substantially different than the ratio of compounds in saliva, suggesting a dominant (but not exclusive) lower airway source of EBC constituents.[9] In oral collections, there is currently no certainty that the oral contribution can be excluded from the sample. In samples collected by endotracheal tube, the immediate source of volatiles and nonvolatiles is the lower airway and lungs (although aspiration of saliva and gastric fluid can contaminate the lower airway fluid).

DILUTION

The ALF component of EBC is highly diluted by condensing vapor phase water. Estimates of the dilution of ALF particles in EBC range from 20-fold to 30,000-fold.[10] A generally accepted number seems to be 2000-fold to 10,000-fold.[11] There may be relevant day-to-day and sample-to-sample intrasubject variability in dilution, although the assays used for assessment of dilution are themselves a source of variability. There is as yet no gold standard dilution marker for EBC. Within a given study, it is worthwhile to standardize against a relevant additional EBC component, such as the conductivity of a lyophilized sample or ion measurements,[10,12] total protein, or urea measurement.[9] Compared with bronchoalveolar lavage, it may be easier to obtain a reliable dilution indicator for EBC because, unlike bronchioalveolar lavage, there is no mechanism by which collection of EBC significantly alters the ALF.[11]

There are 2 times when dilution markers are unnecessary. The first is when multiple biomarkers are measured concurrently and their ratios considered. Ratios among interreactive or biologically related biomarkers can be of particular interest and can eliminate the need for dilution markers. Examples of such ratios include the interferon γ (Th1)/ interleukin (IL) 4 (Th2) ratio,[13,14] nitrite/nitrate (NO_2^-/NO_3^-) ratio,[15] reduced glutathione/oxidized glutathione,[16] and pH (which can be considered a ratio of acids and bases).[17] The second time when dilution markers are unnecessary is when there is a confident assay for a substance that serves as an on-off indicator of an abnormality, such as present–not present. Examples include the presence of *Mycobacterium tuberculosis* DNA (by polymerase chain reaction [PCR]), gastric pepsin,[18,19] rhinovirus RNA (by reverse transcriptase PCR), and anthrax toxin. False-positivity in such assays needs to be nil.

LACK OF GOLD STANDARDS OF LUNG DISEASE ASSESSMENT OR DIAGNOSIS WITH WHICH TO COMPARE EBC MEASUREMENTS

There is currently no gold standard invasive or noninvasive method of determining absolute concentrations of ALF nonvolatile constituents with which EBC can be readily compared. For example, bronchoalveolar lavage is subject to its own dilution concerns. Microsampling techniques that draw fluid from the airway wall by capillary action or suction alter the fluid, creating a lung biomarker equivalent to the Heisenberg Uncertainty Principle. Induced sputum suffers similarly to microsampling techniques in that the fluid expectorated seems to be affected by the sputum production process, at least on subsequent sampling. As a result, there is no consensus as to whether ALF is isotonic, hypotonic, or hypertonic compared with blood. The concentration of sodium ion in the human ALF remains uncertain.

The general disdain for invasive collection of samples from healthy lungs additionally limits or knowledge of normal airway fluid components, and normal variability. The invasiveness or discomfort of collection limits the ability to study airway components. These issues underlie the attractiveness of EBC as a research and clinical tool. The lack of ability to access unadulterated ALF using other means weighs in favor of EBC. EBC has been used to assess the inflammatory effects of sputum induction, which has been shown to increase 2 proinflammatory cytokines, IL6 and tumor necrosis factorα.[20] EBC may be better than other alternatives in assessing the ALF milieu, because it may have fewer drawbacks than other methods.

VALIDATION

EBC is often grouped with exhaled nitric oxide in review articles and insurance company briefings, but, from a validation standpoint, EBC is technically behind exhaled nitric oxide.[1] However, this is not because exhaled NO is a better biomarker than EBC; EBC is not a biomarker at all. Exhaled NO is 1 biomarker, whereas EBC is a matrix in which so many biomarkers have been identified that investigators have not yet been able to concentrate on any 1 of them as they have for exhaled NO. A recent search of PubMed reveals 849 EBC papers, with the first paper in 1979.[21] Publications involving EBC increased greatly at the turn of the century and are still appearing at a significant rate; 70 were published in 2011 and 60 have been published as of June 2012 (**Fig. 1**). These articles cover more than 11 diseases (not including different types of cancers, disease states, and infections) and more than 100 biomarkers, with more being identified monthly. The most common diseases, conditions, and biomarkers are shown in **Figs. 2** and **3**.

COLLECTION OF EBC

As noted earlier, interest in EBC lies mainly with its ease of collection in nearly any setting. EBC can be safely collected orally from spontaneously breathing subjects or from patients undergoing mechanical ventilation.[22–24] The methods of collection for these settings, although simple, vary.

Oral Collection

It takes as little as 1 breath to collect EBC, although, in research practice, longer collection times are often used to ensure that sufficient sample is available for

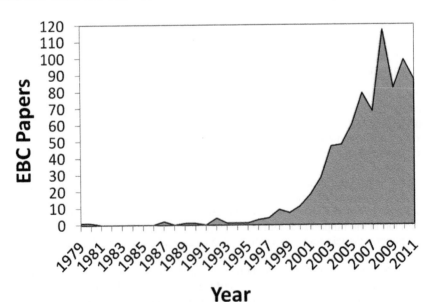

Fig. 1. EBC publications by year in the peer-reviewed literature.

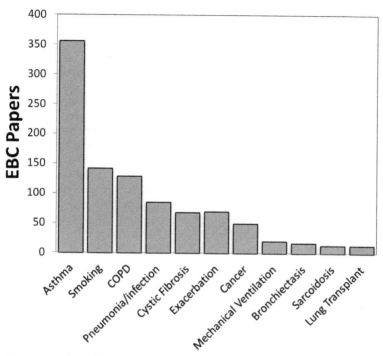

Fig. 2. Common patient diagnoses and conditions reported in EBC publications, including all articles from single studies to reviews. COPD, chronic obstructive pulmonary disease.

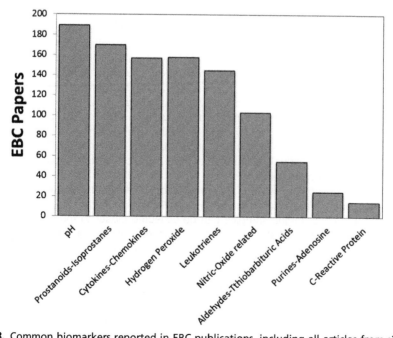

Fig. 3. Common biomarkers reported in EBC publications, including all articles from single studies to reviews.

repeated analysis of multiple biomarkers. Ten minutes of tidal breathing yields 1 to 2 mL of sample, and is well tolerated. Some centers focus on 1 or 2 biomarkers at a time, allowing smaller sample sizes. At our center, the most common oral EBC collection duration is 10 minutes.

Several options exist for collection of EBC samples from both spontaneously breathing and mechanically ventilated patients (**Table 1**). Multiple custom devices have been used throughout the years, using various cooling techniques, device shapes, materials, and coatings. Systems can be made from parts found in respiratory laboratories, and such homemade systems can often be made cheaply, although the expense in terms of personnel time may be substantial. Commercially available equipment is also available. Certain biomarkers are seemingly best collected under set condensation conditions, but these conditions are different for various biomarkers.[11] Although standardized methods of collection and storage for certain individual biomarkers are developing, there is no expectation that there will ever be a standardized EBC collection procedure that will be uniform for all biomarkers. Therefore, any collection method that satisfies the needs of the user and biomarker is acceptable, but there is not, nor should there be, a universal, standardized methodology.

Collection During Mechanical Ventilation

EBC can be collected in as little as 5 minutes during mechanical ventilation but there are several considerations specific to this patient population. The length of time needed to collect an adequate sample depends on the device used for collection (see **Table 1**), the patient (ie, higher volumes of EBC are obtained per given period of time in adults vs neonates), and the humidity devices/settings used (if any) during mechanical ventilation.[24] Samples collected from subjects receiving humidified mechanical ventilation are diluted by the humidified bias flow that travels through the condenser (along with the exhaled breath). Reducing the humidity of the gas delivered to the patient may not be tolerated by the patient and significantly reduces the amount of EBC sample collected over time, but provides less diluted EBC. Dilution of the sample is less likely to affect the measurement of biomarker ratios than specific biomarkers. Another consideration is that EBC collected orally may have different biomarker ranges than EBC collected during mechanical ventilation, because the upper airway is bypassed by the endotracheal or tracheostomy tube. Our group conducted a study of EBC pH before and after intubation and it did not change in healthy subjects[25]; however, the low concentration of ammonia (a base) in endotracheally collected EBC allows EBC pH to be a more sensitive indicator of airway acidification in intubated subjects than in nonintubated subjects.

EBC can be collected 2 ways during mechanical ventilation: in line with the ventilator circuit or at the exhaust port of the ventilator (see **Table 1**). Both methods have pros and cons. In-line samples can be collected closer to the patient (on the expiratory end of the ventilator wye) and is therefore likely to trap larger particles in EBC that may rain out into the ventilator circuit before reaching the exhaust port. Downsides to in-line collection are the need to open the ventilator circuit to place and remove the collection device; this requires interrupting. Also, current in-line collection does not allow analysis of EBC in real time and, depending on the device, may limit the amount of EBC sample that can be collected (typically less than 5 mL). Collection at the exhaust port (postventilator) does not require an interruption of ventilation and can allow continuous collection of EBC and even measurement of EBC pH in real time.[22] Recent technological advances in mechanical ventilation EBC

Table 1
EBC collection systems currently used

EBC Collection System	Manufacturer	Advantages	Disadvantages
ECoScreen I/II	Carefusion, Europe	Most commonly published EBC collection system. More common in European centers. Optional package for determination of total exhaled volume. Has been used to collect EBC during mechanical ventilation	Not readily portable. Cleaning between patients may need to be extensive to abide by standard respiratory care practices. Limited ability to control condensation temperature. No longer distributed in the United States
ECoScreen Turbo	Carefusion, Europe	Lightweight, portable condenser system. Controllable condenser temperature. Disposable collection circuit. Optional package for determination of total exhaled volume	Few publications. No longer distributed in the United States
RTube	Respiratory Research, United States	More total EBC collections performed using RTube than other systems. Multiple collections can be performed concurrently. More common in North American centers. Disposable (no cleaning between patients). Portable. Can be prepared for use in a standard freezer, enabling home collection	Choice and maintenance of set condensing temperature requires optional cooling unit, otherwise condensation temperature is chosen by cooling sleeve preparation temperature and increases during collection
RTube Vent	Respiratory Research, United States	Can be used in line with ventilator circuit or at expiratory port. Insignificant resistance regardless of placement in ventilator circuit	Choice and maintenance of set condensing temperature requires optional cooling unit, otherwise condensation temperature is chosen by cooling sleeve preparation temperature and increases during collection. Few publications (safety data only)
Airway Lining Fluid Analyzer	Respiratory Research, United States	Has both nondisposable and disposable portions. Controllable collection temperature. Collects EBC continuously throughout the course of ventilation. Gas standardizes and measures EBC pH continuously. Compatible with most ventilators	Few publications. Complex system, requires skilled user. Only able to collect EBC at exhaust port of ventilator

collection methods are stimulating this area of EBC research. Certain mechanical ventilators may alter their function in the presence of an EBC collection system, so it is important for a respiratory therapist or other experienced individual to formally assess how the devices interact. Be alert to the effects of any resistance added to the circuit or to the exhaust port.

RANGE OF EBC BIOMARKERS

EBC biomarkers have been categorized (Horvath Task Force[11]), although the categories are open to change. There are several potential categorizations, and biomarkers may be in 1 or more of the following groups:

Categorization group 1
1. Volatile compounds
2. Nonvolatile compounds
3. Nonvolatile compounds derived from volatile compounds

Categorization group 2
4. Very-low-molecular-weight compounds
5. Low-molecular-weight compounds
6. Polypeptides
7. Proteins
8. Nucleic acids

Miscellaneous differentiation
9. Lipid mediators
10. Inorganic molecules
11. Organic molecules
12. Redox relevant molecules
13. pH relevant molecules
14. Cytokines, chemokines

Only a few potentially relevant compounds have so far been reported. Given a sufficiently sensitive assay, it is likely that any stable molecule in the ALF can be found in EBC, and more useful EBC biomarker categories will result from new findings.

The most substantive difference among these categories is between volatile and nonvolatile constituents. Some clearly nonvolatile compounds found in EBC may be derivatives of volatiles. For example, nitrate (NO_3^-) and nitrite (NO_2^-), which are ionized and therefore not volatile, may arise in EBC in part from a reaction of volatile gaseous nitric oxide (NO) after reaction with oxygen.[26] Chloride ion (Cl^-), another nonvolatile, can be at least in part delivered as the volatile hydrochloric acid (HCl).

Volatiles

Volatiles such as acetic acid, formic acid, and ammonia are found in higher concentrations in EBC than nonvolatile constituents, and therefore tend to be easier to measure. Volatile biomarkers may be identified in the high-micromolar or even low millimolar range. Their arrival and concentration in EBC is controlled by different factors than the nonvolatile biomarkers. The amount and size of particles formed by turbulence (or other means) and dilution factors are irrelevant for volatile biomarkers. That dilution markers are not needed may enhance the value of the volatile biomarker assays.

However, other factors are important for interpretation of volatile biomarker levels, including water solubility, gas-liquid partition coefficients, temperature of the source fluid (ALF), temperature of the condenser, pH of the source fluid and EBC, and the opportunity to react within (and therefore be captured by) the EBC matrix or collection device itself. These factors mean that interpretation requires caution. An increased level of formic acid in EBC may not mean more formic acid production in the ALF, but may indicate a lower pH of the ALF (and therefore enhanced volatility because nonvolatile formate ion is protonated in acidic fluid to form the volatile species formic acid). EBC pH as an indicator of ALF pH is important because of acids tend to be volatile from, whereas bases tend to be trapped by, acidic source fluid. When EBC pH is lower than normal, more acid and/or less base has been delivered to and captured in the EBC, primarily because more acid and less base has been volatilized from an acidic airway. Although EBC pH does not equal airway pH, an acidic EBC is created from an acidic airway source fluid, so qualitative noninvasive assessments of airway pH deviation become achievable.

Some of the issues so far determined that should be controlled for when planning to assay volatiles include:

1. Condensation temperature that is sufficiently cold to freeze the EBC may diminish the amount of volatiles (which are more readily absorbed into the liquid phase).[25]
2. Frozen storage may protect reactive or unstable compounds, but may also allow sublimation of the volatiles into the airspace above the frozen EBC (Hunt, personal communication, 2005). These volatiles will be lost when the storage container is opened, unless efforts are made to thaw and remix the sample before opening.
3. Volatile substances respond differently to sample manipulation. Each substance of interest should be studied to control for potential effects of collection duration, temperature, storage conditions, and assay system.

Nonvolatiles

Nonvolatile constituents of EBC make up a broad category containing molecules as small as sodium ion (Na+) and as large as immunoglobulins. There are numerous publications in the literature presenting an individual compound that has been found in EBC (often relying on 1 assay) with levels depending on disease state, with speculation that the biomarker may be valuable in managing the disease of interest. There is optimism, but the more experienced researchers have also learned certain lessons:

1. Confirm the results of your assay with other assays using different methodologies.
2. Ensure that assay controls are performed appropriately and thoroughly; this is perhaps the single most important point for investigators studying EBC. EBC is a highly dilute, low-protein aqueous matrix. If commercially available assay kits for EBC are used, it is important to ensure that the standards used for comparison (standard curve generation) are done in a matrix as similar to that EBC sample as possible. The artifact-producing effect of using improper standards is often called a matrix effect and can be substantial in EBC assays.[27] Using proteinaceous standards (cytokine X in bovine serum albumin), and attempting to compare with unaltered EBC leads to misleading assay values. One choice is for the EBC sample to be altered so as to be substantially similar to the standards (such as by adding albumin). Because of inadequate recognition of matrix effect, it is likely that some of the published data are sufficiently contaminated by artifacts to invalidate their conclusions.
3. The pH of EBC varies in substantially disease states, with pH values as low as 3.5 and has high as 9.0 reported.[17,28] Because the reactivities and stabilities of many of

the other biomarkers of interest are affected by the pH of the fluid in which they are found, and because accuracy of some assays can be affected as well, investigators need to be aware that EBC pH can cause assay artifact as well as loss (or gain) of biomarkers in EBC during storage.

4. In the absence of dilution assessment, different levels of a single EBC biomarker in a disease state may be interpreted either to represent different levels of the biomarker in the ALF or a different amount or size of particles evolved from an otherwise identical ALF. To reiterate an earlier point, ratios among more than 1 related biomarker do not require dilution markers to be of more confident value.

5. Many, if not most, of the nonvolatile constituents found within EBC are identified by assays at the lower limits of their accuracy. Great care should be taken to assure that the assay is reporting correctly, although expectations for assay reproducibility at these low levels are limited. EBC biomarkers have often been criticized as suffering from high intrasubject variability, and therefore being of marginal value. In many cases, this variability may result from assay variability as opposed to biologic or EBC collection system variability. Such assay variability is also found for dilution assessment efforts, which can mathematically compound the overall non-biologic variability and, if not accounted for, can lead to incorrect conclusions, exaggerating the apparent biologic variability or EBC collection system variability.

6. Concentration of EBC samples by lyophilization/dehydration/freeze drying with re-suspension of the lyophilate in small volumes of highly pure water has seemingly allowed for biomarker assessment by immunoassays in the many cases in which the levels were previously too low to be measurable. A 1-mL EBC sample (eg, collected in 7 minutes), can be lyophilized and resuspended in 50 µL, a 20-fold concentration. The advent of multiplex bead arrays has allowed the tiny reconstituted volumes to be used for multiple immunoassays concurrently, opening up an exciting potential, with proof of concept in several studies, to gain a broad window on the balance among cytokines (or other mediators) in the ALF during any respiratory state. The issue of variable dilution remains (unless dilution factors are analyzed), but the ratios among the cytokines are likely to be valid as long as sufficient assay controls have been performed. Cytokines present a particular challenge because, in many cases, they are at the lower limits of detection in serum/plasma and therefore often expected to be at even lower concentrations in EBC. One additional challenge in multiplex cytokine analysis lies in the variation between assay kits, because their ability to detect cytokines varies from one platform to another. The reader is referred to Breen and colleagues[29] (2011) for further information.

A key point is that conscientious assay technique will likely find in EBC any substance of high concentration in the ALF. It is beyond the scope of this article to provide details regarding each of the biomarkers that has been reported in EBC, and new discoveries are being made weekly.

INTERPRETATION OF EBC BIOMARKERS

One of the major challenges in interpreting EBC biomarkers is the difficulty in comparing findings across studies. First, despite EBC methodological recommendations set forth by an American Thoracic Society/European Respiratory Society task force in 2005, many investigators do not fully describe collection methods.[11] Second, there are multiple areas for variation in biomarker assays: (1) differences between laboratories or users, (2) differences between manufacturers or assay kits for the same biomarker, and (3) differences between kit lot numbers from the same manufacturer. This variation makes it difficult to compare biomarker concentrations from 1 study to another. One recommendation is to analyze biomarker trends in terms of relative change rather than absolute concentration. Third, most biomarkers do not have established normal values or ranges. One method to overcome this deficiency is to describe biomarker variations in the context of the individual subject's baseline, so that they serve as their own control. One of the major needs in EBC research is the establishment of methodological standards and normative values specific to each EBC biomarker.

FUTURE OF EBC RESEARCH

With the formation of the International Association for Breath Research (IABR) in 2005, the development of the *Journal of Breath Research* in 2007, and the 2011 Breath Analysis Summit,[30] EBC research is advancing. As EBC research and the resulting literature expand, more methodological studies, reviews, and meta-analyses will be conducted to fully develop EBC science and adequately assess the clinical relevance of EBC biomarkers. Exhaled biomarkers are ideal for many reasons but primarily because they are safe, noninvasive, can be repeatedly measured, and represent the airway milieu. Exhaled breath may reveal more subtle changes in the airway, although it is unknown whether exhaled biomarkers will show disease-induced variations earlier than traditional systemic markers (eg, serum/plasma) and/or pulmonary diagnostics (eg, pulmonary function testing, chest radiograph). Because of the array of biomarkers that can be assessed in exhaled breath, ease of collection, and recent advances in technology, exhaled biomarkers have become an exciting field of research despite methodological issues. Development of sensitive tools for monitoring pulmonary diseases could potentially reduce patient burden, increase patient safety during diagnostic testing, aid in earlier diagnosis, and give pulmonary-specific indicators of disease state, impending infection, and/or treatment effects. Exhaled breath research will expand understanding of pathophysiologic mechanisms underlying pulmonary disease and provide a possible future for development of point-of-care testing. EBC research is an exciting, challenging, and rapidly evolving line of inquiry.

REFERENCES

1. Hunt J. Exhaled breath condensate: an evolving tool for noninvasive evaluation of lung disease. J Allergy Clin Immunol 2002;110(1):28–34.
2. Fairchild CI, Stampfer JF. Particle concentration in exhaled breath. Am Ind Hyg Assoc J 1987;48(11):948–9.
3. Papineni RS, Rosenthal FS. The size distribution of droplets in the exhaled breath of healthy human subjects. J Aerosol Med 1997;10(2):105–16.
4. Tufvesson E, Bjermer L. Methodological improvements for measuring eicosanoids and cytokines in exhaled breath condensate. Respir Med 2006;100(1): 34–8.
5. Zacharasiewicz A, Wilson N, Lex C, et al. Repeatability of sodium and chloride in exhaled breath condensates. Pediatr Pulmonol 2004;37(3):273–5.
6. Sidorenko GI, Zborovskii EI, Levina DI. Surface-active properties of the exhaled air condensate (a new method of studying lung function). Ter Arkh 1980;52(3): 65–8 [in Russian].
7. Gaber F, Acevedo F, Delin I, et al. Saliva is one likely source of leukotriene B4 in exhaled breath condensate. Eur Respir J 2006;28(6):1229–35.

8. Griese M, Noss J, von Bredow C. Protein pattern of exhaled breath condensate and saliva. Proteomics 2002;2(6):690–6.
9. Effros RM, Peterson B, Casaburi R, et al. Epithelial lining fluid solute concentrations in chronic obstructive lung disease patients and normal subjects. J Appl Physiol 2005;99(4):1286–92.
10. Effros RM, Hoagland KW, Bosbous M, et al. Dilution of respiratory solutes in exhaled condensates. Am J Respir Crit Care Med 2002;165(5):663–9.
11. Horvath I, Hunt J, Barnes PJ, et al. Exhaled breath condensate: methodological recommendations and unresolved questions. Eur Respir J 2005;26(3):523–48.
12. Effros RM, Biller J, Foss B, et al. A simple method for estimating respiratory solute dilution in exhaled breath condensates. Am J Respir Crit Care Med 2003;168(12):1500–5.
13. Shahid SK, Kharitonov SA, Wilson NM, et al. Increased interleukin-4 and decreased interferon-gamma in exhaled breath condensate of children with asthma. Am J Respir Crit Care Med 2002;165(9):1290–3.
14. Robroeks CM, Jobsis Q, Damoiseaux JG, et al. Cytokines in exhaled breath condensate of children with asthma and cystic fibrosis. Ann Allergy Asthma Immunol 2006;96(2):349–55.
15. Nguyen TA, Woo-Park J, Hess M, et al. Assaying all of the nitrogen oxides in breath modifies the interpretation of exhaled nitric oxide. Vascul Pharmacol 2005;43(6):379–84.
16. Yeh MY, Burnham EL, Moss M, et al. Non-invasive evaluation of pulmonary glutathione in the exhaled breath condensate of otherwise healthy alcoholics. Respir Med 2008;102(2):248–55.
17. Paget-Brown AO, Ngamtrakulpanit L, Smith A, et al. Normative data for pH of exhaled breath condensate. Chest 2006;129(2):426–30.
18. Samuels TL, Johnston N. Pepsin as a marker of extraesophageal reflux. Ann Otol Rhinol Laryngol 2010;119(3):203–8.
19. Timms C, Thomas PS, Yates DH. Detection of gastro-oesophageal reflux disease (GORD) in patients with obstructive lung disease using exhaled breath profiling. J Breath Res 2012;6(1):016003.
20. Carpagnano GE, Foschino Barbaro MP, Cagnazzo M, et al. Use of exhaled breath condensate in the study of airway inflammation after hypertonic saline solution challenge. Chest 2005;128(5):3159–66.
21. Larson TV, Covert DS, Frank R. A method for continuous measurement of ammonia in respiratory airways. J Appl Physiol 1979;46(3):603–7.
22. Walsh BK, Mackey DJ, Pajewski T, et al. Exhaled-breath condensate pH can be safely and continuously monitored in mechanically ventilated patients. Respir Care 2006;51(10):1125–31.
23. Muller WG, Morini F, Eaton S, et al. Safety and feasibility of exhaled breath condensate collection in ventilated infants and children. Eur Respir J 2006;28(3):479–85.
24. Carter SR, Davis CS, Kovacs EJ. Exhaled breath condensate collection in the mechanically ventilated patient. Respir Med 2012;106(5):601–13.
25. Vaughan J, Ngamtrakulpanit L, Pajewski TN, et al. Exhaled breath condensate pH is a robust and reproducible assay of airway acidity. Eur Respir J 2003;22(6):889–94.
26. Hunt J, Byrns RE, Ignarro LJ, et al. Condensed expirate nitrite as a home marker for acute asthma [letter]. Lancet 1995;346(8984):1235–6.
27. Hom S, Walsh B, Hunt J. Matrix effect in exhaled breath condensate interferon-gamma immunoassay. J Breath Res 2008;2(4):041001.

28. Nicolaou NC, Lowe LA, Murray CS, et al. Exhaled breath condensate pH and childhood asthma: unselected birth cohort study. Am J Respir Crit Care Med 2006;174(3):254–9.
29. Breen EC, Reynolds SM, Cox C, et al. Multisite comparison of high-sensitivity multiplex cytokine assays. Clin Vaccine Immunol 2011;18(8):1229–42.
30. Corradi M, Mutti A. News from the Breath Analysis Summit 2011. J Breath Res 2012;6(2):020201.

Exhaled Breath Condensate pH Assays

Michael D. Davis, BS, RRT[a], John Hunt, MD[b],*

KEYWORDS

- Exhaled breath condensate • Assay • pH • Airway acidification

KEY POINTS

- Exhaled breath condensate (EBC) collection is the only noninvasive method of assessing airway acidity.
- Like all tests, EBC pH is neither perfectly sensitive nor specific for lower airway acidification.
- Acid at any level in the airway can lead to EBC acidification, and an absence of EBC acidification does not exclude the presence of some degree of airway acidification.
- EBC pH assays remain the most successful manner to date to evaluate the role of airway acidification in respiratory disease.

INTRODUCTION

Airway pH is central to the physiologic function and cellular biology of the airway. The causes of airway acidification include (1) hypopharyngeal gastric acid reflux with or without aspiration through the vocal cords, (2) inhalation of acid fog or gas (such as chlorine), and (3) intrinsic airway acidification caused by altered airway pH homeostasis in infectious and inflammatory disease processes.[1] The recognition that relevant airway pH deviations occur in lung diseases is opening doors to new simple and inexpensive therapies.[2,3] This recognition has resulted partly from the ability to use exhaled breath condensate (EBC) as a window on airway acid-base balance, about which data are otherwise difficult or ethically impossible to obtain.

EBC consists primarily of water with trapped aerosolized droplets from the airway lining fluid, and water-soluble volatile compounds. The pH of EBC is determined primarily by the water-soluble volatile gases[4–7] and reflects (but does not precisely quantitate) the pH of airway lining fluid. A low pH value in EBC results from the

Conflict of interest: Dr Davis is supported by grant K99/R00 NR012016 from the National Institute of Nursing Research. Dr Hunt is a cofounder of Respiratory Research, Inc., which manufactures exhaled breath condensate collection equipment. Dr Hunt and the University of Virginia have intellectual property interest in airway pH diagnosis and therapy.
[a] Adult Health and Nursing System, Virginia Commonwealth University, Richmond, 1100 East Leigh Street, Box 980567, VA 23298-0567, USA; [b] Department of Pediatrics, University of Virginia, Box 800386, Charlottesville, VA 22908, USA
* Corresponding author.
E-mail address: Jfh2m@virginia.edu

Immunol Allergy Clin N Am 32 (2012) 377–386
http://dx.doi.org/10.1016/j.iac.2012.06.003
0889-8561/12/$ – see front matter © 2012 Elsevier Inc. All rights reserved.

enhanced volatilization of acids that occurs from an acidic source; in other words, acidic airway lining fluid. Nonvolatile basic anions become protonated within an acidic airway lining fluid and thereby turn into volatile (exhalable) acids. Formic and acetic acid,[7,8] and numerous other acids, join the exhaled airstream when the airway is acidic, are captured by the water condensing in the exhaled breath, and lower the pH of the EBC. In contrast, when the airway lining fluid is alkaline, the ionized conjugate bases of these acids are the dominant species. The ionized conjugate bases are not volatile, and therefore not appreciably exhaled.[6] The association of low airway pH with low EBC pH has been proven empirically with studies of experimental airway acidification in cows.[9] These straightforward concepts have allowed a simple assay (pH), performed on easily collected samples (EBC),[4,10] to provide large amounts of data regarding airway acidity from patients, even in the presence of marked acute airway disease.[11–14]

ADDRESSING THE ARTIFACT OF CARBON DIOXIDE

Most investigators address in some manner the important issue of carbon dioxide (CO_2) affecting the EBC pH. CO_2 is a volatile gas that is a precursor to carbonic acid. CO_2 is not appreciably more volatile from acidic airway lining fluid than from alkaline airway lining fluid. Although CO_2 contributes to the acidity of airway lining fluid, the presence of CO_2 in EBC does not communicate that the airway lining fluid is acidic, because the CO_2 will affect the pH of the EBC regardless of the airway pH. CO_2 leads to substantial EBC acidification if not accounted for in some fashion, and provides noise in the system that limits the ability to identify the smaller effects of the volatile acids, and shrinks the overall effect size of pH measurements in disease by lowering the EBC pH normal range. Gas standardization with either a CO_2-free gas[4,10,15,16] or a gas that contains a known quantity of CO_2[17] seems wise, and has been commonly adopted.

Gas standardization before EBC pH measurement allows samples to be assayed at any time after collection, and clearly improves assay repeatability and overall reproducibility in patient collections.[4,10,15–18] Not all CO_2 is removed through gas standardization via exposing (bubbling) the sample with a CO_2-free gas, partly because the standardizing gas is unlikely to be truly CO_2-free. Overall, however, the levels of CO_2 in EBC are brought to similar low levels for all samples during gas standardization, but some minor effect of residual CO_2 remains.

More recent work from Kullman and Horvath's group[17] in Hungary has raised the possibility that using a known concentration of CO_2 for gas standardizing may improve reproducibility of the assay further. Some loss of effect size between disease and health occurs by so doing, but standardizing on a known concentration of CO_2 may allow for more interlaboratory cooperation. Using CO_2-free gas allows for variable amounts of contaminating CO_2, which, in addition to EBC collection equipment differences, may partly explain why some variability of normal occurs in different laboratories.

It should not be a surprise that the volatile acids trapped in EBC are not as affected by gas standardization procedures as is the CO_2. This finding is simply because CO_2 is a highly volatile gas that is a precursor of an acid, as opposed to being an acid itself, whereas the volatile acids that acidify EBC are trapped by ionization. CO_2 is easy to remove from solution, which likewise removes the carbonic acid that was formed when EBC initially absorbed the CO_2. Thus, the unhelpful effect of exhaled CO_2 on EBC pH is minimized by having the EBC "breathe it back off" during gas standardization.

EBC PH ASSAY VALIDATION AND TECHNICAL ISSUES

The gas standardized EBC pH measurements are substantially reproducible and immune to most potential confounding influences. Compared with other EBC assays, pH is solidly in the range of available assays. Although EBC is a dilute fluid with low ionic strength, pH probes are available that are designed to function even in distilled water. Thus, EBC pH measurement has benefited from the decades of advances in measurement of this standard chemical property. Technological capabilities are readily available to assess concentrations of hydrogen ions as low as 10 fmol/L (which is equivalent to an alkaline pH of 14) and as high as 1 mol/L (an acid pH of 0). Measurement of pH is routinely performed, even in highly purified water such as that used in steam turbines. Measurement of pH of fluids is a well-understood process with no technical hurdles to overcome.

The authors' center has specifically examined and found that the following factors have no effect on the final deaerated EBC pH value: gender, time of day collected, volume of EBC collected, duration of EBC collection, degree of hyperventilation or hypoventilation of the subject, temperature or duration of sample storage, choice of CO_2-free gas used for deaeration (oxygen vs argon), acute use of albuterol/salbutamol by the patient, or methacholine-induced airway obstruction.[4,5,10,19] Age does not seem to be a factor, except in the very elderly, who have a substantially higher incidence of low EBC pH.[20] Although average and median values between races stay consistent, African Americans have been shown to have a higher prevalence of episodes of low pH.[21]

Ammonia is a volatile base that is readily measurable in EBC. Much EBC ammonia seems to be formed in the upper airways through bacterial metabolism of urea.[22] Removal of this oral source of ammonia does not affect EBC pH in healthy adults.[5] However, reasonable evidence exists to support that the ammonia reduces the sensitivity of EBC pH to airway acidity. Oral ammonia neutralizes CO_2 initially, and also exhaled acids that are relevant to airway acidity, lessening the ability of the exhaled acids to lower EBC pH. As a result, orally collected EBC pH in lung diseases is less likely to be acidic than EBC collected from endotracheally intubated patients. However, in healthy patients, the values of orally versus endotracheally collected samples are similar.[4] This loss of sensitivity to acidic airways of orally collected EBC samples seems to prevent the EBC pH measurement from being overly sensitive in the primary clinical indication for its measurement (discussed later).

Condenser temperature does seem to affect EBC pH during collection. In healthy subjects (without breath acidification), the authors found no difference in EBC pH at collection temperatures of −56°C to room temperature. However, in subjects with acidic breath, collecting at condenser temperatures low enough to cause sample freezing is found to lead to less capture of exhaled acids (which cannot go into solution into ice, after all). Thus the authors always perform EBC collection at temperatures that do not allow sample freezing during collection.

An additional effect on pH arises during sample storage while frozen. The authors have noted that, after freezing a stored sample with low pH, if the sample container is opened before thawing, the measured pH of the sample is higher than the initial measurement. These observations are consistent with sublimation from the solid EBC of relevant volatile acids, a conclusion supported by the ability to prevent this artifact from occurring by allowing the sample to thaw and shaking the container before opening it. The authors strongly recommend this approach.

EBC pH can be affected by duration of gas standardization and temperature during measurement. Although earlier investigators recommended a bubbling time of 7 to 12 minutes to achieve CO_2 standardization,[4,15–17] more recent studies show stabilization occurring in as few as 1 to 5 minutes.[18,23] Recent studies have also shown that sample temperature may cause artifact in EBC pH[24] consistent with temperature's well-known effects on pH. This finding suggests that in some circumstances, more careful control for sample temperature may be desirable.

A final technical comment regarding EBC pH measurement seems warranted. Not all pH probes are appropriate for measurement in the low ionic strength matrix of EBC. Certain technologies simply will not function. The authors have found that Ross-type pH probes are uniformly effective, and standard glass probes with a substantial leak of internal fluid are generally effective. Before selecting a probe, the authors confirm that it calibrates in low ionic strength pH buffers identically to the standard pH buffers, and that addition of ionic strength adjusters/enhancers to samples of EBC does not affect the pH readings provided by the probe. These two tests help assure that the probe is not adversely functioning in the low ionic strength EBC.

NORMAL EBC PH VALUES

Normal values of gas-standardized (CO_2-free) EBC pH have been reported from multiple investigators and range between 7.5 and 8.1.[4,10,11,16,19,21,25–33] In the authors' normative database from 404 subjects, the mean pH was 7.83 and the median pH was 8.0.[19] The bell curve data distribution cuts off at a pH of approximately 7.4, with a scattering of values below that level that are clearly not part of the normal distribution. EBC pH values below 7.4 occur in 6% of this population. These values likely represent subjects with airway acidification that may be transiently symptomatic or asymptomatic, and may result from proximal acid reflux or from temporary innate immune responses against viral infections. Based on these data and data from more than 10,000 samples collected or analyzed in the laboratory, the authors consider pH values less than 7.4 to be abnormal.

There are potential confounders of the EBC pH levels. The authors have found that substantial intake of ethyl alcohol to the point of inebriation may modestly lower EBC pH. This finding may reflect alcohol's metabolism to acetic acid, which when exhaled can then alter EBC pH. It also may reflect alcohol-induced augmentation of gastroesophageal reflux to the laryngeal level.[25] Additionally, recent smoking, oral ingestion of food or beverages, and particularly ingestion of fluids[6,34,35] with volatile acids (vinegar) within 20 minutes of EBC collection may cause substantial artifact, with a lower EBC pH.[6,34,35] The authors' protocol for providing an EBC sample for pH assay includes that nothing except water should be ingested for 30 minutes before collection.

ANATOMIC SOURCE OF THE DETERMINANTS OF EBC PH

It is reasonable to assume that any significant acidification of the airway lining fluid that is exposed to the exhaled airstream will add acid to EBC. In patients who are endotracheally intubated, pharyngeal contribution will be nil. As part of the airway, the oropharynx likely can contribute to EBC pH when the sample is collected orally,[15] but it does not in general have a strong effect. In keeping with this, salivary pH and EBC pH do not correlate,[4] and pH of EBC samples collected through oral breathing are the same as those collected subsequently from the endotracheal tube after intubation in patients undergoing elective surgery.[4] Therefore, intentional profound experimental acidification of the pharynx can lead to temporary EBC acidification.[25] This finding reflects the ability of EBC pH assays to identify the presence of a source fluid, at any airway level, sufficiently acidic to protonate certain bases to their volatile conjugate acids.

Although the mouth can contribute to the acidity of EBC, it also contributes to alkalinization of EBC through ammonia (NH_3), which is a volatile base produced in high concentrations in the mouth and lungs of many people and often is the highest-concentration substance measurable in EBC.[5] Initial speculation about NH_3 controlling EBC pH was forwarded,[22] prompting studies to collect the empiric evidence that has allowed for an improved understanding of the role of NH_3. Several interesting observations have been made regarding oral ammonia. First, removing the potential oral ammonia contribution to EBC through bypassing the mouth with endotracheal intubation does not affect the EBC pH in healthy subjects.[4] Second, removing ammonia (likely along with other volatiles) from EBC through lyophilization and resuspension does not affect EBC pH.[5] Third, it is uncommon to have a low EBC pH value without a low NH_3 level in EBC; however, it is common to find low NH_3 levels with normal EBC pH levels.[5] These observations led to the current understanding that high oral production of NH_3 can blunt the EBC pH signal of volatile acids coming from the lungs, and thereby decrease the sensitivity of orally collected EBC pH assays to identify lung acidification. However, when the acids exhaled from the airway are sufficient to overcome the modest neutralizing effect of oral NH_3, a low EBC pH signal represents low airway lining fluid pH. An additional, albeit less confident notion is that minor differences in EBC pH values between groups within the pH range that is considered normal are of uncertain meaning.

Extensive data have now been collected from intubated humans showing that EBC pH is low in disease states.[12] Recently, a study performed in 12 patients showed that an endobronchially intubated healthy lung produces an EBC that is alkaline, whereas when the contralateral tuberculosis-infected lung destined for excision is included in the EBC sampling, the values are acidic.[13] These data provide invasive measurements necessary to help prove that acidification of the lower airways does occur and, as one would expect, is heterogeneous, with pH low in the sick portions of the lung.

RESEARCH AND CLINICAL UTILITY OF EBC PH MEASUREMENTS

EBC pH is now perhaps the most commonly performed EBC assay, probably for two reasons. Foremost is that investigators realize that airway pH deviation is a particularly relevant pathologic process that affects almost every other aspect of lung disease that may interest them. One cannot ignore such a core component of how the airways and lungs function. Secondly, the pH assay is easy to perform.

The relevance of EBC pH and what it reflects—airway pH—is important to reiterate. Airway acidification is not just a biomarker of inflammation. Rather, airway acidification seems to be a central pathologic process in its own right that results in multiple broadly important adverse effects. Airway acidity leads to inflammation (neutrophilic and eosinophilic), bronchospasm, bronchial hyperreactivity, ciliary dysfunction, epithelial dysfunction, augmented oxidative damage, abnormal fluid transport, inhibition of transport of cationic drugs such as albuterol, and alteration of cellular death pathways, including inhibition of apoptosis.[1] Airway pH is entirely relevant to almost any project undertaken by an airway researcher. The authors now believe that cell and molecular biology research into airway and lung diseases risks yielding substantially incorrect conclusions if the researchers fail to take into account the disease-associated deviations in pH from normal that are likely present. How can one ascertain what normal neutrophil apoptosis rate is in patients with chronic obstructive pulmonary disease (COPD) when the cells on the bench are only incubated at neutral pH, yet the airway pH in disease may be pronouncedly acidic?

Unlike most other assays in EBC, no value of pH exists that is "undetectable." However, this is misleading; pH measurement represents a net proton concentration signal resulting from amounts and ratios of multiple acids and bases within the EBC. A "normal" EBC pH may mean that no volatile acids are present (which can therefore be interpreted as "undetectable"), or it may mean that volatile bases from an alkaline mouth or alkaline proximal airway have neutralized the volatile acids arising from an acidic area in the distal airway (thereby suggesting that EBC pH has relevant limitations to its sensitivity, similar to other EBC assays). A low EBC pH can confidently be said to result from a low airway lining fluid pH at some level. However a normal EBC pH does not exclude the presence of airway acidification, unless little NH_3 is present in the EBC also.

Undoubtedly some published results have suffered from unrecognized deficiencies of pH probes, effects of freeze-sublimation that artifactually raises EBC pH, and excessively cold condenser temperatures. Most likely more technological validations remain to be undertaken, but the field has advanced well, and application of this assay to provide outcome measures in large clinical studies and to assist in clinical patient management is now a reasonable consideration.

Continuous EBC pH Monitoring in Intubated Patients

A system was developed by Respiratory Research, Inc. (a University of Virginia faculty–owned company of which the corresponding author is a director) and the United States Air Force that allows for measurement of EBC pH continuously. Known as the ALFA monitor, this system condenses breath from the expiratory port of mechanical ventilators, performs gas standardization at two levels using hospital wall oxygen supplies, and measures, displays, and records the EBC pH in digital and graphical formats. Because of the time delay for condensation and processing, the result is a second-to-second recording of an EBC pH moving average representing EBC production from the lungs during the previous 5 to 10 minutes. To date, the authors have performed continuous pH condensimetry on more than 250 humans, ranging from neonates to the elderly, for as long as 70 days uninterrupted. With the oropharynx eliminated as a source of volatile acids, this system allows for selective measurement of lung acidity. In the absence of oral NH_3 contribution, the EBC pH becomes a higher-sensitivity assay for airway acidity.

Diseases for which the authors have continuous pH condensimetry anecdotal data revealing lung acidification include acute asthma, cystic fibrosis, COPD, infection with respiratory syncytial virus, acute respiratory disease syndrome (ARDS), and bronchopulmonary dysplasia. In these disease processes, pH changes gradually over hours to days. An EBC pH greater than 7.4 is commonly associated with relative lung health, and pH levels associated with disease fall within the 4.0 to 6.0 range,[12] similar to those found in oral EBC collections from healthy and ill patients, respectively.[10] In unpublished data, the authors have observed frequent gradual decline in EBC pH during general anesthesia, which is currently of uncertain significance. Additionally, they have observed drastic pH fluctuations after witnessed aspiration events (**Fig. 1**).

This technology is functioning for research to study time course of pH changes in the airways. Currently, knowing that the airway lining fluid pH is abnormally low may be only prognostically valuable, because no approved therapeutic is clinically available for neutralizing acidic airway pH. But airway pH modifying therapies are being tested,[3] and when available will create a desire to know what the airway pH is in a given patient so that these airway pH–modifying therapies can be used appropriately.

Assessing for Acid Reflux–Induced Respiratory Symptoms

Initially, the authors and others considered that acid reflux could confound EBC pH assays and prevent the gaining of insights into airway pH. However, with time, they have realized that the airways can acidify intrinsically or extrinsically, with the extrinsic pathways being inhalation of acid gases and aspiration of acid reflux. When considering factors that confound, acid reflux is at the top of the list, because it confounds or complicates every respiratory illness. Acid reflux is perhaps the most diagnostically

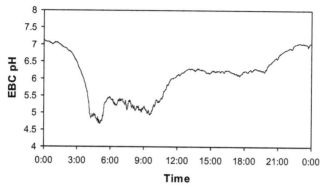

Fig. 1. Twenty-four-hour ALFA monitor continuous breath pH condensimetry tracing of a neonatal patient. Note the sudden pH decrease followed by slow recovery to baseline over the subsequent 12 hours. The drop corresponded with a sudden increase in respiratory support needs accompanied by suctioning of formula from the endotracheal tube.

frustrating entity in pulmonary medicine, because (1) the diagnostics are invasive and not designed or validated for use in respiratory system indications (eg, esophageal pH probes, which use normal reference ranges relevant to esophageal disease but irrelevant to aspiration disease) and (2) it is so common.

EBC pH offers a noninvasive assessment of airway pH that can be performed repeatedly. For example, transient acidification of the breath associated with chronic cough seems to be an excellent indicator that the cough will respond to acid blockade therapy with proton pump inhibitors (PPIs). The authors' studies have shown that patients whose cough symptoms decreased with PPI use invariably had transient breath acidification, and those whose cough failed to respond had no breath acidification (**Fig. 2**). These findings provide a novel method to determine which patients with asthma or COPD have confounding acid reflux without resorting to expensive and indefinite (and commonly indeterminate) PPI empiric trials.

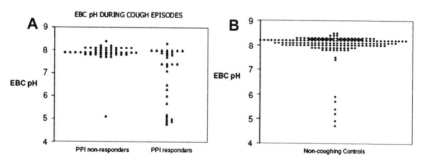

Fig. 2. EBC pH values (A) from patients whose chronic cough did and did not respond to proton pump inhibition (PPI) and (B) from noncoughing controls. Note that multiple samples were collected from each patient, with all data plotted as individual samples. Approximately 50% of the EBC samples from PPI-responsive coughers had low pH values. Note that all patients whose symptoms responded had at least one episode of breath acidification during four to eight breath collections collected at the time of cough. (*Adapted from* Hunt J, Yu Y, Burns J, et al. Identification of acid reflux cough using serial assays of exhaled breath condensate pH. Cough 2006;2:3; with permission.)

Studies of Lung Diseases in Spontaneously Breathing Subjects

The initial purpose for which the authors developed the EBC pH assay was to open a window onto lung chemistry, with pH a centrally involved characteristic. The results of their work and of others using the EBC pH assay has provided the strongest support to date that the airways become acidified in numerous respiratory disorders. The EBC pH assay, although not perfect, has undergone validation and vetting internationally. It is also the assay that has the most published technical validation data supporting the technique.[15] The authors currently believe that EBC pH decline is most relevant in the settings of acute asthma exacerbations, COPD, and acute lung injury and ARDS (representing intrinsic airway acidification), and for assessing gastric acid aspiration in the settings of chronic cough, asthma, COPD, lung transplant rejection, pulmonary fibrosis, vocal cord dysfunction, and exercise-induced dyspnea/bronchospasm. This purpose may be the most immediately valuable from a patient point of view, because therapies exist to help reflux-induced symptoms if a diagnosis is made.

SUMMARY

EBC is the only convenient, noninvasive, ethically acceptable method of assessing airway acidity that is currently available, especially for repeated sampling in acutely ill patients. Like all tests, EBC pH is neither perfectly sensitive nor specific for lower airway acidification. Many of the validation issues have been adequately addressed. The data must be interpreted cautiously, because acid at any level in the airway can lead to EBC acidification, and an absence of EBC acidification does not exclude the presence of some degree of airway acidification. EBC pH measurements remain the most successful method to evaluate the role of airway acidification in respiratory disease.

REFERENCES

1. Ricciardolo FL, Gaston B, Hunt J. Acid stress in the pathology of asthma. J Allergy Clin Immunol 2004;113:610–9.
2. Shin HW, Shelley DA, Henderson EM, et al. Airway nitric oxide release is reduced following phosphate buffered saline inhalation in asthma. J Appl Physiol 2007; 102:1028–33.
3. Davis MD, Paget-Brown A, Dwyer ST, et al. Safety and therapeutic potential of inhaled alkaline glycine in obstructive airway disease [abstract]. Respir Care 2012;56.
4. Vaughan J, Ngamtrakulpanit L, Pajewski TN, et al. Exhaled breath condensate pH is a robust and reproducible assay of airway acidity. Eur Respir J 2003;22:889–94.
5. Wells K, Vaughan J, Pajewski TN, et al. Exhaled breath condensate pH assays are not influenced by oral ammonia. Thorax 2005;60:27–31.
6. Rothe MB, Siemers G, Decker RM. The pH-value of exhaled breath condensate - mainly influenced by exhaled volatile compounds. Eur Respir J 2005;26:2405.
7. Vaughan JW, Gaston B, MacDonald T, et al. Acetic acid contributes to exhaled breath condensate acidity in asthma [abstract]. Eur Respir J 2001;18:P3083.
8. Greenwald R, Ferdinands JM, Teague WG. Ionic determinants of exhaled breath condensate pH before and after exercise in adolescent athletes. Pediatr Pulmonol 2009;44:768–77.
9. Bunyan D, Smith A, Davidson W, et al. Correlation of exhaled breath condensate pH with invasively measured airway pH in the cow. Eur Respir J 2005;26:2407.
10. Hunt JF, Fang K, Malik R, et al. Endogenous airway acidification. Implications for asthma pathophysiology. Am J Respir Crit Care Med 2000;161:694–9.

11. Gessner C, Hammerschmidt S, Kuhn H, et al. Exhaled breath condensate acidification in acute lung injury. Respir Med 2003;97:1188–94.
12. Walsh BK, Mackey DJ, Pajewski T, et al. Exhaled-breath condensate pH can be safely and continuously monitored in mechanically ventilated patients. Respir Care 2006;51:1125–31.
13. Skrahina T, Smirnou A, Astrauko A, et al. Separate lung exhaled breath condensate collection confirms intrapulmonary origin of exhaled breath condensate acidification [abstract]. Eur Respir J 2007;30:365S.
14. Carter SR, Davis CS, Kovacs EJ. Exhaled breath condensate collection in the mechanically ventilated patient. Respir Med 2012;106:601–13.
15. Horvath I, Hunt J, Barnes PJ. Exhaled breath condensate: methodological recommendations and unresolved questions. Eur Respir J 2005;26:523–48.
16. Borrill ZL, Smith JA, Naylor J, et al. The effect of gas standardisation on exhaled breath condensate pH. Eur Respir J 2006;28:251–2.
17. Kullmann T, Barta I, Lazar Z, et al. Exhaled breath condensate pH standardised for CO_2 partial pressure. Eur Respir J 2007;29:496–501.
18. Lin JL, Bonnichsen MH, Thomas PS. Standardization of exhaled breath condensate: effects of different de-aeration protocols on pH and $H(2)O(2)$ concentrations. J Breath Res 2011;5:011001.
19. Paget-Brown AO, Ngamtrakulpanit L, Smith A, et al. Normative data for pH of exhaled breath condensate. Chest 2006;129:426–30.
20. Cruz MJ, Sanchez-Vidaurre S, Romero PV, et al. Impact of age on pH, 8-isoprostane, and nitrogen oxides in exhaled breath condensate. Chest 2009;135:462–7.
21. Hauswirth DW, Sundy JS, Mervin-Blake S, et al. Normative values for exhaled breath condensate pH and its relationship to exhaled nitric oxide in healthy African Americans. J Allergy Clin Immunol 2008;122:101–6.
22. Effros RM. Do low exhaled condensate NH4+ concentrations in asthma reflect reduced pulmonary production? Am J Respir Crit Care Med 2003;167:91.
23. Prieto L, Orosa B, Barato D, et al. The effect of different periods of argon deaeration on exhaled breath condensate pH. J Asthma 2011;48:319–23.
24. Koczulla AR, Noeske S, Herr C, et al. Ambient temperature impacts on pH of exhaled breath condensate. Respirology 2010;15:155–9.
25. Hunt J, Yu Y, Burns J, et al. Identification of acid reflux cough using serial assays of exhaled breath condensate pH. Cough 2006;2:3.
26. Brunetti L, Francavilla R, Tesse R, et al. Exhaled breath condensate pH measurement in children with asthma, allergic rhinitis and atopic dermatitis. Pediatr Allergy Immunol 2006;17:422–7.
27. Carpagnano GE, Barnes PJ, Francis J, et al. Breath condensate pH in children with cystic fibrosis and asthma: a new noninvasive marker of airway inflammation? Chest 2004;125:2005–10.
28. Carraro S, Folesani G, Corradi M, et al. Acid-base equilibrium in exhaled breath condensate of allergic asthmatic children. Allergy 2005;60:476–81.
29. Kostikas K, Papatheodorou G, Ganas K, et al. pH in expired breath condensate of patients with inflammatory airway diseases. Am J Respir Crit Care Med 2002;165:1364–70.
30. Nicolaou NC, Lowe LA, Murray CS, et al. Exhaled breath condensate pH and childhood asthma: unselected birth cohort study. Am J Respir Crit Care Med 2006;174:254–9.
31. Niimi A, Nguyen LT, Usmani O, et al. Reduced pH and chloride levels in exhaled breath condensate of patients with chronic cough. Thorax 2004;59:608–12.

32. Rosias PP, Dompeling E, Dentener MA, et al. Childhood asthma: exhaled markers of airway inflammation, asthma control score, and lung function tests. Pediatr Pulmonol 2004;38:107–14.

33. Varnai VM, Ljubicic A, Prester L, et al. Exhaled breath condensate pH in adult Croatian population without respiratory disorders: how healthy a population should be to provide normative data? Arh Hig Rada Toksikol 2009;60:87–97.

34. Kullmann T, Barta I, Antus B, et al. Drinking influences exhaled breath condensate acidity. Lung 2008;186:263–8.

35. Calusic AL, Varnai VM, Macan J. Acute effects of smoking and food consumption on breath condensate pH in healthy adults. Exp Lung Res 2011;37:92–100.

Asthma Biomarkers in Sputum

Joseph D. Spahn, MD[a,b,c,d,*]

KEYWORDS

• Asthma • Biomarker • Sputum • Airway

KEY POINTS

- Sputum eosinophilia has consistently been found to predict worsening of asthma control with inhaled glucocorticoid dose reduction.
- Sputum can be used to aid in the diagnosis of asthma and in the task of distinguishing asthma from chronic obstructive pulmonary disease in patients who present with evidence for fixed airflow obstruction.
- Inhaled glucocorticoid therapy can be titrated upward or downward with the goal of keeping the sputum eosinophil count at or less than 2%.

Airway inflammation plays an important role in the pathogenesis of asthma. Several inflammatory cells are thought to contribute. Among these, the eosinophil seems to be a major effector cell. Studies using bronchoscopy with bronchoalveolar lavage and/or biopsy have consistently found airway eosinophilia in subjects with asthma. In addition, airway eosinophilia has consistently been shown to correlate with asthma symptoms, diminished lung function, and airway heightened responsiveness (AHR). As such, there has been great interest in developing easily performed and noninvasive markers of eosinophilic inflammation that can be used in the diagnosis and management of asthma.

Although great progress has been made, there remains no gold standard noninvasive measure of airway inflammation. In the past decade, exhaled nitric oxide (eNO) and induced sputum have been advocated as sensitive and noninvasive measures of airway inflammation. Much of the pioneering work to develop sputum induction as a practical tool to evaluate airway inflammation has come from Hargreave and colleagues at the Firestone Institute for Respiratory Health at McMaster University

[a] Ira J. and Jacqueline Neimark Laboratory of Clinical Pharmacology in Pediatrics, National Jewish Health, 1400 Jackson Street, Denver, CO 80206, USA; [b] Division of Pediatric Clinical Pharmacology, Department of Pediatrics, National Jewish Health, 1400 Jackson Street (J312), Denver, CO 80206, USA; [c] Division of Allergy-Clinical Immunology, Department of Pediatrics, National Jewish Health, 1400 Jackson Street (J312), Denver, CO 80206, USA; [d] Department of Pediatrics, University of Colorado Health Sciences Center, Denver, CO, USA
* Division of Pediatric Clinical Pharmacology, Department of Pediatrics, National Jewish Health, 1400 Jackson Street (J312), Denver, CO 80206.
E-mail address: katialr@njhealth.org

Immunol Allergy Clin N Am 32 (2012) 387–399
http://dx.doi.org/10.1016/j.iac.2012.06.004
0889-8561/12/$ – see front matter © 2012 Elsevier Inc. All rights reserved.

in Hamilton, Ontario, Canada. For more information on the development and practical aspects of performing sputum induction, the reader is referred to comprehensive reviews on this topic.[1,2]

Following therapeutic intervention, sputum induction is the only practical and direct way to measure repeatedly the many cellular and molecular indices of inflammation involved in asthma in large numbers of patients. Other measures, such as eNO, provide indirect evidence for eosinophilic inflammation, whereas bronchoscopy is invasive, expensive, and difficult to perform in large numbers of patients. This article focuses on the clinical usefulness of sputum eosinophil counts in asthma.

SPUTUM EOSINOPHILIA AS A DIAGNOSTIC AID FOR ASTHMA

Asthma can be difficult to diagnose because it is characterized by such symptoms as wheezing, shortness of breath, and cough that fluctuate in severity and frequency. The bases of diagnosis, in addition to symptoms, are variable airflow limitations measured by a 12% or more improvement in forced expiratory volume in 1 second (FEV_1) after β-agonist administration, or the presence of AHR as measured by methacholine or histamine challenge. However, many subjects with asthma have normal lung function and lack a significant bronchodilator response. As a result, β-agonist response lacks sufficient sensitivity as a screening tool for asthma. Methacholine challenges have good sensitivity and specificity, but they are not routinely performed because of the technical expertise, the significant expense, and the time required to administer the procedure. As a result of these various difficulties in diagnosing asthma, interest has emerged in determining the usefulness of noninvasive measures of eosinophilic inflammation in making the diagnosis of asthma.

A recent study from Smith and colleagues[3] compared the clinical usefulness of sputum eosinophilia and eNO with peak expiratory flow (PEF) variability, baseline FEV_1, and FEV_1/forced-vital-capacity (FVC) ratio, and change in FEV_1 following an oral glucocorticoid course in making the diagnosis of asthma in adults with symptoms that suggest asthma. Forty-seven adults who presented to the clinic with symptoms that suggested asthma were enrolled to undergo spirometry, before albuterol, after albuterol, and after a course of oral glucocorticoids, methacholine challenge, and serial PEF measures. In addition, the subjects underwent sputum induction and eNO analysis. Of the 47 subjects, 17 (36%) were diagnosed with asthma based on a positive β-agonist response ($\geq$12%) improvement in FEV_1 following albuterol inhalation or positive methacholine challenge. Both eNO and sputum eosinophilia had sensitivities and specificities that were superior to other conventional measures, such as baseline FEV_1 or FEV_1/FVC ratio, peak flow variability, or change in FEV_1 following a steroid course. Sputum eosinophilia ($\geq$3%) had the highest sensitivity (86%) and specificity (88%) of the measures studied, suggesting that it is superior to all other conventional measures for making the diagnosis of asthma.

Sputum induction can also be useful in determining whether a subject with fixed airflow obstruction has evidence for eosinophilic versus neutrophilic inflammation. Determining the type of inflammation has important clinical implications, as described in a study published by Fabbri and colleagues.[4] These investigators sought to determine whether patients with fixed airflow obstruction had distinct pathologic and functional characteristics that stemmed from a history of asthma or chronic obstructive pulmonary disease (COPD). Forty-six patients who presented to the clinic with fixed airflow obstruction underwent lung function studies, eNO and sputum analysis, high-resolution chest computed tomography (CT) scans, and bronchoscopy with lavage and biopsy. Twenty-seven had a history of COPD, whereas the remaining 19 had a history of asthma. Both groups had similar degrees of obstruction with FEV_1 values of 56% predicted, and similar levels of AHR. Patients with a history of asthma had significantly more eosinophils in their peripheral blood, sputum, bronchoalveolar lavage, and airway mucosa. In addition, they had higher eNO levels and higher diffusion capacities, and had lower residual volumes and lower CT scan emphysema scores. In addition, asthmatics had fewer neutrophils in their sputum and bronchoalveolar lavage fluid compared with subjects with COPD.

As expected, asthmatics were more likely to have eosinophilic inflammation and higher eNO levels. In contrast, patients with COPD secondary to tobacco smoking had a neutrophil predominance. Thus, 2 distinct pathophysiologic processes can result in the same outcome of fixed airflow obstruction. It is important to distinguish between the 2 processes because patients with fixed airflow limitation and eosinophilia are more likely to respond to glucocorticoids than those with neutrophilia. As such, asthmatics with fixed airflow obstruction should not be labeled as having COPD, and are likely to derive benefit from asthma medications. Methacholine responsiveness and lung function measures were not able distinguish between the 2 types of lung disease, whereas the presence of airway eosinophilia was. Thus, sputum induction with cell differential can be used to direct appropriate therapy in patients with fixed airflow limitation.

SPUTUM EOSINOPHILIA AND ASTHMA SEVERITY

A large study from the United Kingdom sought to evaluate how asthma severity based on lung function impairment and symptom frequency relates to several noninvasive measures of airway inflammation. The study involved 74 adults with varying levels of asthma, from mild intermittent to severe persistent asthma, and 22 nonatopic controls.[5] The investigators evaluated induced sputum indices, such as total numbers of inflammatory cells, eosinophils, neutrophils, and basophils, and mediators of inflammation, such as eosinophil cationic protein, myeloperoxidase, and tryptase, in addition to spirometry, PEF variability, daily symptom scores, and responsiveness to methacholine. Significant correlations were noted between sputum eosinophil counts, eosinophil cationic protein levels, and asthma severity with regard to FEV_1, symptoms, PEF variability, and methacholine responsiveness. In addition, severe asthmatics had the highest sputum eosinophil counts, despite the use of high-dose inhaled glucocorticoid and, in some patients, chronic oral glucocorticoid therapy, with values 19 to 44 times higher than values noted among the nonatopic, nonasthmatic controls. The investigators concluded that sputum eosinophilia and increased sputum eosinophil cationic protein levels significantly correlate with increasing asthma severity, and eosinophilic inflammation persists despite aggressive glucocorticoid therapy in patients with severe asthma.

By performing a multivariate regression analysis of 205 asthmatics who underwent induced sputum induction for entry into clinical studies, Woodruff and colleagues[6] examined the relationships among sputum eosinophil counts, sputum neutrophil counts, FEV_1 values, and methacholine provocation concentration (PC) of methacholine or histamine causing a 20% drop in FEV_1 after controlling for confounding factors (PC20). Forty percent of the subjects were on an inhaled glucocorticoid and 45% had FEV_1 values of less than 80% of predicted. The investigators found 4 factors to be significant confounders of the relationship between cellular inflammation and airway function: age, sex, ethnicity, and inhaled glucocorticoid use. After controlling for these factors, an inverse relationship between sputum eosinophil counts and FEV_1 and PC20 values was noted. The higher the sputum eosinophil count, the lower the

FEV$_1$ and PC20 values. Sputum neutrophils were also inversely correlated with FEV$_1$ but not with PC20 values. The investigators concluded that both eosinophils and neutrophils contribute to airway caliber, but only eosinophilia is associated with bronchial hyperresponsiveness. There was also a relationship between inhaled glucocorticoid use and sputum eosinophils counts, whereas no such association was noted between sputum neutrophils and inhaled glucocorticoid use.

This is among the largest studies evaluating the relationship between sputum inflammatory cells and asthma severity. Because of the large number of subjects, multivariate analyses could be performed. After controlling for several confounding variables, airway eosinophilia was strongly associated with reduced lung function and greater AHR, whereas airway neutrophilia was associated only with reduced lung function. The finding that neutrophilia was associated with diminished lung function but not related to inhaled glucocorticoid therapy argues against inhaled glucocorticoids being an effective modality in patients with neutrophilic inflammation. As such, therapies directed specifically at neutrophils may prove most useful in improving airway caliber in asthmatics with neutrophilic, as opposed to eosinophilic, inflammation. This issue is addressed in greater detail later.

Romagnoli and colleagues[7] conducted a study to determine whether eosinophilic inflammation contributes to poor asthma control and asthma severity. Nineteen subjects with poorly controlled asthma, 16 subjects with well-controlled asthma, and 8 nonasthmatic control subjects were studied. In addition, 23 subjects were classified as having mild to moderate asthma, 14 of whom were poorly controlled, whereas 12 were classified as having severe persistent asthma, 5 of whom were poorly controlled. Sputum eosinophil, leukotriene E4, eosinophil cationic protein, and RANTES (regulated on activation in normal T cells, expressed and secreted protein) levels were increased in subjects with poorly controlled compared with those with well-controlled asthma, whereas no differences in sputum eosinophil levels or any of the inflammatory markers studied were noted among the various levels of asthma severity. This study confirmed a relationship between asthma control and airway eosinophilia that is independent of asthma severity. In addition, it showed that some patients with severe asthma have ongoing eosinophilic inflammation despite glucocorticoid therapy. The presence of sputum eosinophilia in this group of patients should prompt the physician to further investigate adherence with glucocorticoid therapy. If adherence is thought to be adequate, consideration of alternative immunomodulator therapy should be made.

Airway inflammation is thought to be present in children with asthma, but until recently there were few published studies to support this claim. In one of the earliest studies evaluating airway inflammation in childhood asthma, Cai and colleagues[8] measured lung function and performed sputum induction in 50 asthmatic and 72 healthy children. Data were available from 42 asthmatic children. Of these, 15 were asymptomatic, 16 had active asthma, and 11 had a recent exacerbation of their asthma. All of the asthmatic children were on inhaled glucocorticoids at the time of evaluation. The healthy children had little evidence for inflammation, with few sputum eosinophils and epithelial cells (0.3% and 1.5% respectively) noted, whereas the asthmatic children had significantly greater percentages of eosinophils (4.3%) and epithelial cells (14%). Among the asthmatics, the investigators found an inverse relationship between lung function and sputum eosinophils, and a trend toward higher eosinophil counts among asthmatics with active disease.

This was among the first published studies in children with asthma showing eosinophilic inflammation and association with epithelial damage. It suggests that, as is the case for adult asthmatics, eosinophils play a prominent role in the pathogenesis of childhood asthma. The finding of increased numbers of epithelial cells in the sputum supports the concept that eosinophils are involved in the damage to the airway epithelium, a feature that has been consistently noted in subjects with asthma.

In one of the largest studies evaluating airway inflammation in children with asthma published to date, Covar and colleagues[9] performed sputum induction in 117 subjects on completion of a 5-year study evaluating the efficacy of budesonide and nedocromil compared with placebo and following a washout period of 2 to 4 months. Sputum induction was successful in 90 of 117 subjects on completion of the study and in 74 of 90 subjects after a washout period of 2 to 4 months. Reasons for failed induction included inadequate sample volume, presence of more than 80% squamous cells, and inability to tolerate the hypertonic saline inhalation for a sufficient period of time. The investigators found the budesonide-treated subjects to have significantly fewer sputum eosinophils compared with the subjects treated with placebo and nedocromil. Subjects with sputum eosinophilia at study discontinuation were more likely to have worsening asthma control requiring a rescue course of prednisone during the washout period. In addition, sputum eosinophilia was associated with increased eNO levels, atopy, greater β-agonist reversibility, and greater asthma severity during the treatment period.

This study shows the advantages and disadvantages of sputum induction in children with asthma. Sputum induction was successful in most children. In addition, it provided valuable information for evaluating the effect of chronic inhaled glucocorticoid use on reducing airway inflammation and the association between sputum eosinophilia and asthma severity and control. More importantly, sputum induction showed that patients with eosinophilia at treatment discontinuation were at greatest risk of having an asthma relapse. However, only 63% of subjects were able to perform 2 successful sputum inductions. This observation suggests that serial sputum eosinophil measures are not as useful as other noninvasive measures of inflammation, such as eNO. In addition, the investigators found that a minority of subjects (8%) developed significant bronchospasm (mean decrease in FEV_1, 30.4%) despite pretreatment with 360 mcg of albuterol. The children who developed bronchospasm had lower baseline lung function, greater disease severity, and greater β-agonist reversibility compared with children who tolerated sputum induction. The investigators concluded that sputum induction can provide information on eosinophilic inflammation and treatment response. However, they also said that sputum induction will likely remain a research tool because of the time and technical expertise required.

Sputum induction has also been performed in children presenting to the emergency department with acute asthma. Gibson and colleagues[10] obtained sputum by nebulized normal saline or spontaneous expectoration in 37 of 42 children (mean age 12 years) presenting to the emergency department with acute asthma. The mean FEV_1 of the children at entry was 59% of predicted, and 62% subsequently required hospitalization. Sputum eosinophilia was found in 78%. That is, 43% of the subjects had pure eosinophilia, whereas 35% had combined eosinophilia and neutrophilia. Eosinophilia was more likely in children not on a controller agent and in those with the greatest degree of airflow limitation. The pattern of airway inflammation (noneosinophilic, eosinophilic, and combined eosinophilic and neutrophilic) was not related to onset of exacerbation. Thus, in children presenting to the emergency department with acute asthma, eosinophilia is present in most cases and is related to the severity of the exacerbation. In addition, those with neutrophilic inflammation were not more likely to have a rapid onset to their exacerbation.

EFFECT OF INHALED GLUCOCORTICOID ON SPUTUM EOSINOPHILS

Several studies have evaluated the effect of inhaled glucocorticoids on airway inflammation assessed by sputum induction. Most have shown significant reductions in eosinophilia following inhaled glucocorticoid therapy. The question of whether salmeterol has antiinflammatory effects was addressed by Currie and colleagues,[11] who evaluated the effects of fluticasone-salmeterol combination therapy on airway inflammation in patients with moderate persistent asthma. Before entry, all subjects were well controlled on inhaled glucocorticoid therapy alone. Inhaled glucocorticoid therapy was then discontinued, and the subjects were treated with a 4-week course of salmeterol. Spirometry was performed, airway hyperresponsiveness was assessed, and measurements were taken of eNO, sputum and circulating blood eosinophils, and sputum/serum eosinophil cationic protein levels following the 1-month course of salmeterol therapy and following 2 weeks of twice-daily fluticasone 100 mg administered in combination with salmeterol. The addition of low-dose fluticasone to salmeterol resulted in significant reductions in sputum (4.3-fold) and blood eosinophils (1.3-fold), eNO (1.8-fold), and sputum eosinophil cationic protein (2.2-fold) levels compared with treatment with salmeterol alone. In addition, significant improvements in FEV_1 and airway hyperresponsiveness were noted following the addition of fluticasone to salmeterol.

This study shows the effectiveness of inhaled glucocorticoids in suppressing airway inflammation while improving lung function and reducing airway hyperresponsiveness. In addition, it indirectly addresses the issues raised regarding the long-term safety of long-acting β-agonists.[12] Several indices of airway inflammation significantly decreased following the addition of low-dose fluticasone in patients treated with salmeterol alone for 4 weeks, suggesting that salmeterol has little if any antiinflammatory effects. This study's major flaw stems from the investigators' failure to measure airway inflammation before discontinuing inhaled glucocorticoid therapy. Had measures of inflammation been performed at that point, they could have determined the magnitude of the change in airway inflammation following the substitution of an inhaled glucocorticoid with the long-acting β-agonist, salmeterol. Even so, this study supports the current recommendations that long-acting β-agonists be used only in combination with an inhaled glucocorticoid.[13,14]

The question of how rapidly inhaled glucocorticoids act in reducing airway inflammation was addressed by Gibson and colleagues.[15] Forty-one adult asthmatics underwent baseline sputum induction. The 26 subjects with sputum eosinophilia (defined as sputum eosinophil count of R7%) were enrolled in a randomized, crossover study to receive 2400 mg of budesonide or placebo on 2 separate study days. Symptoms, lung function, airway hyperresponsiveness, and sputum induction were then measured 6 hours after therapy. Compared with placebo, use of budesonide resulted in a substantial reduction in sputum eosinophils (25% vs 37%; $P = .05$) and a 2.2-fold improvement in AHR, whereas no changes in lung function, symptoms, apoptotic eosinophils, or sputum mast cells were noted.

The investigators had hypothesized that budesonide would result in a rapid reduction in eosinophils by inducing eosinophil apoptosis. Apoptosis, or programmed cell death, is an important way the body safely rids itself of cells, such as eosinophils, that contain toxic compounds. In vitro studies found glucocorticoids to induce eosinophil apoptosis, thus induction of apoptosis seemed to be the most likely mechanism of action. Although budesonide was associated with a rapid reduction in airway eosinophils, apoptosis was not the mechanism for the observed reduction. The investigators postulated that the reduction in sputum eosinophils was the result of vascular exudation and cell adhesion. A large dose of budesonide resulted in a rapid reduction in sputum eosinophils. This study did not address the question of how rapidly improvements in asthma symptoms and lung function follow the reduction in sputum eosinophils.

SPUTUM EOSINOPHILIA AS A PREDICTOR FOR RESPONSE TO GLUCOCORTICOIDS

In the past half-dozen years, it has become increasingly clear that not all asthmatics display a favorable response to inhaled glucocorticoid therapy. Among the many possible predictors of glucocorticoid response that have been evaluated, sputum eosinophils have consistently been found to be the best predictors. Pavord and colleagues[16] were among the first to report that subjects with asthma and sputum eosinophilia were likely to respond to inhaled glucocorticoid therapy, whereas those without eosinophilia were not. They studied the effect of a 2-month course of budesonide (400 mg) administered twice daily in 23 subjects with asthma previously treated with short-acting β-agonists alone. Eosinophilia, defined as a sputum eosinophil count of 3% or more, was noted in 14 of 23 subjects (61%) at baseline. The eosinophilic and noneosinophilic groups had similar baseline FEV_1 values, FEV_1/FVC values, and symptom scores, whereas the eosinophilic subjects were more likely to be atopic and to have a greater degree of AHR at baseline. Following treatment with budesonide, the eosinophilic subjects had a greater improvement in AHR and reduction in symptom scores compared with the noneosinophilic subjects. Even though this study was small and not placebo controlled, it provided valuable insight into the usefulness of sputum induction in assessing response to inhaled glucocorticoid therapy.

Similar findings have been observed regarding response to oral glucocorticoid therapy, as shown by Little and colleagues.[17] Thirty-seven moderate persistent asthmatics with compromised lung function (FEV_1 76% of predicted) and treatment with inhaled glucocorticoids (median dose 800 mg/d beclomethasone dipropionate [BDP] or equivalent) underwent eNO and induced sputum measurements before and after a 14-day course of prednisolone. At baseline, 32% of the subjects had an increased eNO level (O10 ppb) and 37% had sputum eosinophilia (O4%). The investigators found that both increased sputum eosinophils and eNO treatment predicted improvement in lung function following a 2-week course of prednisone. Eighty-three percent of the subjects with an eNO value of greater than 10 ppb had greater than a 15% improvement in their FEV_1 (positive predictive value [PPV] of 83%), whereas the PPV for sputum eosinophilia was 64%. By combining both eNO and sputum eosinophil count, the PPV remained high at 72%, whereas the negative predictive value significantly increased to 79%. Thus, increased levels of both eNO and sputum eosinophilia were associated with a good response to prednisolone, whereas low levels of the 2 markers were associated with a poor response to a short course of prednisolone.

The National Heart, Lung, and Blood Institute's Asthma Clinical Research Network used eNO and sputum eosinophils to determine the relative beneficial and systemic effects of inhaled glucocorticoids.[18] Thirty adult asthmatics (FEV_1 at baseline 74% of predicted) received escalating doses of either fluticasone propionate (FP) (88, 353, and 704 mg/d) or BDP (168, 672, and 1344 mg/d) in an open-label parallel trial. Primary efficacy measures included improvement in FEV_1 and reduction in AHR, whereas systemic effect was measured by overnight plasma cortisol suppression. Maximal lung function improvement occurred at the lowest dose of FP studied (88 mg/d), whereas a larger dose of BDP (672 mg/d) was required. For methacholine response, larger doses of both compounds were required to achieve maximal effect.

As expected, both inhaled glucocorticoids produced a dose-dependent suppression of overnight plasma cortisol production.

The investigators noted a wide range of steroid response, with some patients having no response, whereas others displayed large improvements in both lung function and AHR. Subjects most likely to have a significant improvement in lung function were more likely to have increased eNO levels, a greater degree of β-agonist reversibility, and a lower FEV_1/FVC ratio at baseline. In contrast, those who displayed a significant improvement in AHR were more likely to have sputum eosinophilia.

Although limited by small sample size, this study contributes several important clinical points. First, it remains among the few studies to compare, in a single study, both the efficacy and systemic effect of inhaled glucocorticoids. Second, it shows the steep dose-response curve for improvement in FEV_1 for potent inhaled glucocorticoids, such as FP, with maximal improvement in FEV_1 occurring at the lowest dose studied. Third, although maximal efficacy occurred early in the dose-response curve, no such plateau exists with regard to systemic effects: the higher the inhaled glucocorticoid dose, the greater the systemic effects. Fourth, individuals with low eNO levels and no sputum eosinophils were unlikely to favorably respond to FP or BDP regardless of the dose studied. Fifth, increased eNO levels predicted a favorable change in lung function, whereas airway eosinophilia predicted a favorable reduction in AHR.

Not all studies have shown lack of steroid responsiveness in noneosinophilic asthmatics, as shown in a study by Godon and colleagues,[19] who sought to determine (1) the prevalence of sputum eosinophilia in poorly controlled asthma, and (2) whether response to inhaled glucocorticoid depended on sputum eosinophilia. Fifty-one steroid-naive asthmatics performed spirometry, methacholine challenges, and sputum induction at baseline and following 1-month of treatment with FP 250 mg twice daily or placebo. At baseline, 71% had sputum eosinophilia with a mean sputum eosinophil count of 9.1%, whereas 29% had no sputum eosinophils. Other than the marked difference in sputum eosinophils, there were no clinical or lung function differences between the 2 groups. The noneosinophilic and eosinophilic groups responded equally well to the 1-month course of fluticasone with improvements in symptoms, lung function, and PC20 values noted.

Several aspects of this study are worth discussing. First, nearly one-third of the subjects with poorly controlled asthma had a sputum eosinophil counts of less than 1%, and nearly half (45%) had sputum eosinophil counts of less than 3%. If eosinophils play an essential role in poor asthma control, what is the driving force of the poor control in the noneosinophilic subjects? In addition, why were inhaled glucocorticoids effective in the noneosinophilic subjects, especially given the large number of studies that failed to show efficacy of inhaled glucocorticoid therapy in noneosinophilic asthma? These questions speak to the complexity of asthma. Not only eosinophils but many cell types and mediators of inflammation contribute to asthma pathogenesis. Thus, it is unlikely that a single mediator or inflammatory cell will provide all of the information needed to assess an individual's level of asthma control and response to therapy.

SPUTUM EOSINOPHILIA AS A PREDICTOR OF ASTHMA RELAPSE

Although it is widely thought that increasing eosinophilic airway inflammation results in worsening asthma, little has been published on this issue. Jatakanon and colleagues[20] studied whether airway inflammation increases in subjects who develop an acute asthma exacerbation as a result of tapering of inhaled glucocorticoid doses. Fifteen well-controlled asthmatics on inhaled glucocorticoid therapy (O800 mg/d) had their dose decreased to 200 mg/d. Serial spirometry, induced sputum, eNO measurements, and methacholine challenges were performed every 2 weeks for 8 weeks. Reduction in inhaled glucocorticoid therapy resulted in asthma worsening in nearly 50% of the subjects. Those who developed an exacerbation had a significantly greater number of sputum eosinophils (13.6% vs 0.2%) at entry into the study and before inhaled glucocorticoid reduction, whereas no differences were noted with respect to lung function, bronchial hyperresponsiveness, or eNO levels. The investigators also noted significant increases in both sputum eosinophils and eNO levels in the patients who developed an exacerbation, whereas no change in these markers of inflammation was observed in those who remained stable despite a significant reduction in inhaled glucocorticoid therapy. The change in eNO level and sputum eosinophils correlated with reductions in lung function. In addition, using multiple regression analysis, the investigators found a change in the sputum eosinophil count following reduction in inhaled glucocorticoid dose to be the best predictor of loss of asthma control.

This study addresses the relationship between increasing airway inflammation and the development of an asthma exacerbation. Airway eosinophilia was the only risk factor that predicted those at risk of developing worsening asthma control following a reduction in inhaled glucocorticoid therapy. Despite significant eosinophilia at baseline in subjects who developed an acute exacerbation with inhaled glucocorticoid dose reduction, their eNO levels were not increased. This observation has been previously noted and is a limitation to monitoring eNO levels in patents on inhaled glucocorticoids. The clinical implications of this study are that sputum eosinophilia in the presence of inhaled glucocorticoid therapy precludes any attempt at tapering the inhaled glucocorticoid dose. Whether the dose of inhaled glucocorticoid should be increased in these patients is another question that needs to be studied.

In a similarly designed study, Leuppi and colleagues[21] sought to determine predictors for failed reduction of inhaled glucocorticoids in 50 adult asthmatics well controlled on inhaled glucocorticoid therapy. With inhaled dose reduction, 78% of the subjects had an exacerbation of their asthma, whereas 14% were able to tolerate a complete reduction of their inhaled glucocorticoid dose. Significant predictors of an asthma exacerbation following inhaled glucocorticoid taper included the presence of AHR to both mannitol and histamine, the development of responsiveness to mannitol during the inhaled glucocorticoid reduction phase, and increased sputum eosinophils at the penultimate inhaled glucocorticoid dose preceding the failed inhaled glucocorticoid dose reduction. Neither symptoms, spirometry, nor eNO levels predicted an asthma exacerbation with inhaled glucocorticoid dose reduction.

In another study, Jones and colleagues[22] compared the usefulness of eNO with sputum eosinophils and AHR in predicting loss of asthma control (LOAC) following inhaled glucocorticoid withdrawal in 78 subjects with mild to moderate asthma controlled on inhaled glucocorticoid therapy. Eighty percent of the subjects developed LOAC during inhaled glucocorticoid withdrawal with significant correlations noted between LOAC and changes in eNO and symptoms, FEV_1, sputum eosinophils, and AHR. In addition, the PPVs for predicting and diagnosing LOAC for eNO, sputum eosinophils, and AHR were all similar. In subjects who developed LOAC, the mean FEV_1 decreased 11.9%, mean eNO level increased from 9.67 to 20.5 ppb in those who developed LOAC (a 2.16-fold increase), and sputum eosinophils increased 4.73-fold.

The question of whether sputum eosinophilia could predict worsening asthma control in children has not been as thoroughly studied. Zacharasiewicz and colleagues[23] recently had 40 well-controlled asthmatic children undergo titration of their inhaled glucocorticoid dose by 50% every 8 weeks until an exacerbation developed or the inhaled glucocorticoid was completely withdrawn. Spirometry, AHR testing, eNO, sputum eosinophils, and exhaled breath condensate collection occurred at each visit and were used to predict success or failure of inhaled glucocorticoid dose reduction. Seventy-five percent of children tolerated at least 1 dose reduction and in 30% inhaled glucocorticoid therapy was discontinued. The absence of sputum eosinophils before inhaled glucocorticoid titration predicted a successful inhaled glucocorticoid taper. In the 38% of children who developed an asthma exacerbation, the mean sputum eosinophil count increased from 0.5% to 15.5% and eNO levels increased from 16 to 53 ppb. None of the mediators of inflammation collected in exhaled breath condensate were useful in predicting an acute asthma exacerbation following inhaled glucocorticoid withdrawal. Using a multiple logistic regression, only increased sputum eosinophils were significant predictors of a failed inhaled glucocorticoid reduction.

In summary, sputum eosinophilia has consistently been found to predict worsening of asthma control with inhaled glucocorticoid dose reduction. Increased sputum eosinophils before reduction nearly always predicted LOAC. In addition, increasing sputum eosinophils during sequential inhaled glucocorticoid dose reduction also predicted subsequent LOAC. Sputum induction could conceivably be performed just once before initiating inhaled glucocorticoid withdrawal, or serially as the dosage is reduced. If the asthmatic had an increased eosinophil count at baseline, inhaled glucocorticoid reduction would not be advised. However, if eosinophil count were not increased, careful reduction could proceed with the taper halted at the first sign of increasing eosinophilic inflammation.

EOSINOPHILIA AND ASTHMA MANAGEMENT

Treatment decisions in asthma are now made largely from symptoms and simple measures of lung function, such as PEF or FEV_1. Whether measures of airway inflammation and AHR are more useful than symptoms and lung function in the management of asthma has been a topic of intense interest.[24–27] Following the publication of the study by Sont and colleagues[24] in 1999, in which assessment of AHR was superior to symptoms and lung function assessment in achieving optimal asthma, other parameters have been studied, including eNO[25] and sputum eosinophils.[26,27]

Green and colleagues[26] were the first to determine whether a management strategy that minimized sputum eosinophils was more effective than a standard management strategy for reducing asthma exacerbations. Seventy-four adults with moderate to severe asthma were enrolled in a 1-year study in which they were randomly selected to receive standard asthma management based on symptom frequency and lung function impairment or asthma management based on normalization of sputum eosinophils and symptom reduction. After 1 year, there were fewer severe exacerbations (35 vs 109) and fewer hospitalizations (1 vs 6) in the sputum management group versus those in the standard management group. There was no difference in the dose of inhaled glucocorticoid used between the 2 groups during the course of the study. The investigators concluded that a treatment strategy designed to normalize sputum eosinophils might reduce severe asthma exacerbations without the need for additional antiinflammatory medications.

This study suggests that management of asthma by normalizing airway eosinophils may be superior to management of asthma based on symptoms and lung function. This approach is appealing if asthma is thought to be a disease mediated by airway inflammation. Titrating medications up or down based on the extent of eosinophilic inflammation makes more intuitive sense than using indirect measures of inflammation, such as symptoms and lung function. The study by Sont and colleagues[24] titrated medications based on the level of bronchial hyperresponsiveness and found this approach to be superior to that using symptoms and lung function in guiding therapy. However, the improvement in outcome parameters in that study came at the expense of higher doses of inhaled glucocorticoids.

A more recent and revealing study by Jayaram and colleagues[27] evaluated the effectiveness of sputum cell counts in guiding asthma management with the primary goal of reducing exacerbations. A total of 117 subjects were enrolled into a randomized, parallel group study of 2 treatment strategies over a 2-year period. The clinical strategy used symptoms and spirometry to guide treatment, whereas the sputum strategy was intended to keep sputum eosinophil counts at 2% or less. The primary outcome was relative risk reduction for occurrence of the first asthma exacerbation and time to first exacerbation. Secondary outcomes included the type and severity of exacerbation and cumulative dose of inhaled glucocorticoid during the study. There were 126 exacerbations, with significantly fewer exacerbations in the sputum strategy (37%) versus the clinical strategy group (63%). The time to first exacerbation was also longer and the number of subjects requiring prednisone was lower in the sputum strategy compared with the time and number in the clinical strategy group. In the 102 exacerbations in which sputum was obtained before treatment, 70% were noneosinophilic. The reduction in exacerbations in the sputum strategy group came solely from reduction in eosinophilic exacerbations, which accounted for approximately one-third of all exacerbations. In addition, the cumulative dose of inhaled glucocorticoid was similar between the 2 groups.

This study supports and extends the findings noted by Green and colleagues[26]: by adjusting therapy to keep sputum eosinophil counts at 2% or less, the number of acute asthma exacerbations in patients with moderate and severe persistent asthma can be reduced. The most novel finding from the present study was the observation that most exacerbations could not be prevented even by monitoring sputum eosinophil counts because eosinophilia was present in only 30% of the exacerbations. The investigators raise the important clinical question of how noneosinophilic exacerbations should be treated. As discussed earlier, several studies have failed to show that inhaled glucocorticoids are effective in noneosinophilic asthmatics. The investigators suggest that current treatment is merely palliative, and that the exacerbation must resolve spontaneously or with antibiotic therapy if a bacterial infection is present. These data are likely to change how acute asthma is understood and managed, especially if sputum induction becomes more common in its management.

SUMMARY

In the past decade, a large number of studies have shown the clinical usefulness of induced sputum. Although induced sputum may not be as easily and quickly performed as eNO, it can provide a greater amount of information regarding the cellular and molecular processes involved in asthma and other obstructive pulmonary diseases. Induced sputum can be used to aid in the diagnosis of asthma and in the task of distinguishing asthma from COPD in patients who present with evidence for fixed airflow obstruction. Several studies have shown sputum eosinophils to be associated with both asthma severity and level of asthma control. In addition, the presence of sputum eosinophilia strongly predicts a favorable response to glucocorticoid therapy. In contrast, the absence of sputum eosinophilia predicts a poor response to glucocorticoid therapy. Sputum eosinophilia also predicts asthma relapse in subjects who have their inhaled glucocorticoid reduced or withdrawn. Inhaled glucocorticoid therapy can be titrated upward or downward with the goal of keeping the sputum eosinophil count at or less than 2%. By effectively treating sputum eosinophilia, the number of asthma exacerbations can be significantly reduced compared with managing asthma based on symptoms and lung function.

REFERENCES

1. Pavord ID, Pizzichini MM, Pizzichini E, et al. The use of induced sputum to investigate airway inflammation. Thorax 1997;52:498–501.
2. Belda J, Leigh R, Parameswaran K, et al. Induced sputum cell counts in healthy adults. Am J Respir Crit Care Med 2000;161:475–8.
3. Smith AD, Cowan JO, Filsell S, et al. Diagnosing asthma: comparison between exhaled nitric oxide measurements and conventional tests. Am J Respir Crit Care Med 2004;169:473–8.
4. Fabbri LM, Romagnoli M, Corbetta L, et al. Differences in airway inflammation in patients with fixed airflow obstruction due to asthma or chronic obstructive pulmonary disease. Am J Respir Crit Care Med 2003;167:418–24.
5. Louis R, Lau LC, Bron AO, et al. The relationship between airways inflammation and asthma severity. Am J Respir Crit Care Med 2000;161:9–16.
6. Woodruff PG, Khashayar R, Lazarus SC, et al. Relationship between airway inflammation, hyperresponsiveness, and obstruction in asthma. J Allergy Clin Immunol 2001;108:753–8.
7. Romagnoli M, Vachier P, Tarodo de la Fuente P, et al. Eosinophilic inflammation in sputum of poorly controlled asthmatics. Eur Respir J 2002;20:1370–7.
8. Cai Y, Carty K, Henry RL, et al. Persistence of sputum eosinophilia in children with controlled asthma when compared with healthy children. Eur Respir J 1998;11: 848–53.
9. Covar RA, Spahn JD, Martin RJ, et al. Safety and application of induced sputum analysis in childhood asthma. J Allergy Clin Immunol 2004;114:575–82.
10. Gibson PG, Norzila MZ, Fakes K, et al. Pattern of airway inflammation and its determinants in children with acute severe asthma. Pediatr Pulmonol 1999;28:261–70.
11. Currie GP, Syme-Grant NJ, McFarlane LC, et al. Effects of low dose fluticasone/salmeterol combination on surrogate inflammatory markers in moderate persistent asthma. Allergy 2003;58:602–7.
12. Nelson HS, Weiss ST, Bleecker ER, et al. The Salmeterol Multicenter Asthma Research Trial. A comparison of usual pharmacotherapy for asthma or usual pharmacotherapy plus salmeterol. Chest 2006;129:15–26.
13. National Asthma Education and Prevention Program. Expert panel report: guidelines for the diagnosis and management of asthma update on selected topics–2002. J Allergy Clin Immunol 2002;110:S141–219.
14. 2006 GINA report: global strategy for asthma management and prevention. 2006. Available at: www.ginasthma.org. Accessed January 18, 2006.
15. Gibson PG, Saltos N, Fakes K. Acute anti-inflammatory effects of inhaled budesonide in asthma: a randomized controlled trial. Am J Respir Crit Care Med 2001;163:32–6.
16. Pavord ID, Brightling CE, Woltmann G, et al. Non-eosinophilic corticosteroid unresponsive asthma. Lancet 1999;353:2213–4.
17. Little SA, Chalmers GW, MacLeod KJ, et al. Non-invasive markers of airway inflammation as predictors of oral steroid responsiveness in asthma. Thorax 2000;55: 232–4.
18. Szefler SJ, Martin RJ, King TS, et al. Significant variability in response to inhaled corticosteroids for persistent asthma. J Allergy Clin Immunol 2002;109:410–8.

19. Godon P, Boulet LP, Malo JL, et al. Assessment and evaluation of symptomatic steroid-naive asthmatics without sputum eosinophilia and their response to inhaled corticosteroids. Eur Respir J 2002;20:1364–9.
20. Jatakanon A, Lim S, Barnes PJ. Changes in sputum eosinophils predict loss of asthma control. Am J Respir Crit Care Med 2000;161:64–72.
21. Leuppi JD, Salome CM, Jenkins CR, et al. Predictive markers of asthma exacerbation during stepwise dose reduction of inhaled corticosteroids. Am J Respir Crit Care Med 2001;163:406–12.
22. Jones SL, Kittelson J, Cowan JO, et al. The predictive value of exhaled nitric oxide measurements in assessing changes in asthma control. Am J Respir Crit Care Med 2001;164:738–43.
23. Zacharasiewicz A, Wilson N, Lex C, et al. Clinical use of noninvasive measurements of airway inflammation in steroid reduction in children. Am J Respir Crit Care Med 2005;171:1077–82.
24. Sont JK, Luuk N, Willems A, et al. Clinical control and histopathologic outcomes of asthma when using airway hyperresponsiveness as an additional guide to long-term treatment. Am J Respir Crit Care Med 1999;159:1043–51.
25. Smith AD, Cowan JO, Brassett KP, et al. Use of exhaled nitric oxide to guide treatment in chronic asthma. N Engl J Med 2005;352:2163–73.
26. Green RH, Brightling CE, McKenna S, et al. Asthma exacerbations and sputum eosinophil counts: a randomized controlled trial. Lancet 2002;360:1715–21.
27. Jayaram L, Pizzichini MM, Cook RJ, et al. Determining asthma treatment by monitoring sputum cell counts: effect on exacerbations. Eur Respir J 2006;27:483–94.

Tissue-Based and Bronchoalveolar Lavage–Based Biomarkers in Asthma

Sally E. Wenzel, MD

KEYWORDS

• Tissue-based biomarkers • Bronchoalveolar lavage–based biomarkers • Asthma

KEY POINTS

- There are no tissue or bronchoalveolar lavage biomarkers that are specific for asthma in general.
- A biomarker is defined as a cell or compound of interest that has been measured in at least 2 different studies, which is associated with disease, its severity, phenotype, or a specific process associated with that disease.
- Recent efforts to phenotype asthma are strongly linked with the evolution of biomarkers specific to that phenotype.

INTRODUCTION

Asthma is increasingly understood to be a disease consisting of multiple different phenotypes. This heterogeneous disease presents a diagnostic and treatment challenge, especially in moderate to severe asthmatics who continue to be poorly controlled despite high-dose systemic or inhaled steroids. It is likely that previous studies, which have not accounted for this heterogeneity, have limited the ability to identify single biomarkers. As of 2012, there are no tissue or bronchoalveolar lavage (BAL) biomarkers that are specific for asthma in general. In this article, tissue and BAL biomarkers of asthma are evaluated from their use in asthma in the context of the phenotype that they may best represent. For purposes of this article, a biomarker is defined as a cell or compound of interest that has been measured in at least 2 different studies, which is associated with disease, its severity, phenotype, or a specific process (forced expiratory volume in 1 second) associated with that disease. It is hoped that studies that better link biomarkers to specific phenotypes will eventually improve the ability to evaluate genetic features, diagnose, measure progression, and tailor treatments. Although some biomarkers may only be associated

Division of Pulmonary Allergy and Critical Care Medicine, Department of Medicine, Asthma Institute, University of Pittsburgh Medical Center, Northwest 931 Montefiore Hospital, 3459 Fifth Avenue, Pittsburgh, PA 15213, USA
E-mail address: wenzelse@upmc.edu

Immunol Allergy Clin N Am 32 (2012) 401–411
http://dx.doi.org/10.1016/j.iac.2012.06.011
0889-8561/12/$ – see front matter © 2012 Elsevier Inc. All rights reserved.

with disease, it is also likely that some may be mechanistically involved. Some of these biomarkers may then also become targets for specific treatment.

BIOMARKERS FOR EOSINOPHILIC ASTHMA

Tissue eosinophils have been studied in the greatest detail and most studies support that eosinophils in the tissue are generally increased in asthma (**Table 1**).[1] For many years, it was believed that eosinophils were a specific biomarker for asthma, but more recently, many studies using tissue and sputum samples have shown that eosinophils are present only in a percentage of patients with asthma, with estimates between 40% and 60% of asthmatics.[2-4] This situation has led to an increasingly accepted concept that asthma, defined as reversible airflow limitation or bronchial hyperresponsiveness with accompanying clinical symptoms, can be divided into those with and without eosinophils. Eosinophils are a biomarker of the eosinophilic phenotype. This phenotype seems to identify a group of patients with more symptomatic disease, more risk of exacerbations, and, in patients with severe asthma, a higher risk of near fatal events. Only a few tissue studies have sorted patients with asthma by their eosinophil numbers and no longitudinal studies have evaluated the change in tissue eosinophils over time. Several published studies have compared tissue and BAL eosinophils; however, a recent study found modest concordance between biopsy and sputum eosinophils, with sputum identifying more eosinophilic patients.[5] Because bronchoscopy is never likely to be performed at short intervals in patients, or in relation to exacerbations, the prospective ability of tissue eosinophils to guide and monitor therapy is limited. However, sputum eosinophilia seems to be a reasonable surrogate.[6,7]

In severe asthma, the presence of tissue eosinophils has been extensively evaluated in a cross-sectional manner. In this subgroup, there is persistent eosinophilia in tissue despite high-dose oral and inhaled steroids. At least 1 study suggested that tissue eosinophilia is more prevalent in late-onset rather than early-onset disease, consistent with the greater likelihood for aspirin-sensitive (or related hypereosinophilic) subtypes of asthma to occur later in life.[3,8] However, persistent tissue eosinophilia can be seen in asthma that begins at any age. In the tissue, the eosinophilic phenotype has been defined as those patients with tissue eosinophils greater than 2 times the standard deviation of the mean number measured in normal individuals.[2,3,9]

Considerable effort has been spent to identify factors that contribute to the tissue eosinophils. However, few studies have consistently observed relationships between tissue cytokine, chemokine, or lipid mediator levels and eosinophils. Only one of these factors, interleukin 5 (IL-5), has been specifically inhibited in humans and shown to lower tissue eosinophil levels.[10] IL-5 plays a crucial role in eosinophil recruitment,

Table 1	
Biomarkers associated with phenotypic types or aspects of asthma	
Phenotypes	**Biomarkers**
Eosinophils	IL-4, IL-5, IL-13, eotaxins, 15-HETE, 15-LO, CysLTs
Neutrophils	IL-8, LTB4, MMP-9
Paucigranulocytic	Smooth muscle, mast cells in smooth muscle
Remodeling	SBM, collagens, tenascin, TGF-β, chymase-positive mast cells

Abbreviations: CycLT, cysteinyl leukotrienes; HETE, hyroxyeicosetetrenoic acid; IL, interleukin; LO, lipoxygenase; MMP, matrix metalloproteinase; SBM, subepithelial basement membrane; TGF, transforming growth factor.

expansion, and survival in numerous murine models of asthma.[11,12] In addition, it promotes differentiation of eosinophil precursors in the bone marrow. During eosinophil development, there is upregulation of the IL-5 receptor on CD34+ cells and this population increases in bone marrow, blood, and sputum 24 hours after inhaled allergen challenge.[13,14] A recent study reported that 10 mg of inhaled IL-5 had no effect on tissue eosinophils of asthmatics, but in normal individuals, a significant increase in tissue eosinophils occurred. Despite the lack of increase in tissue eosinophils, there was a dramatic decrease in eosinophil progenitor cells in the asthmatic but not in normal individuals. The reasons for these differences are not clear.[15] IL-5 has also been shown to increase in BAL fluid after segmental allergen challenge, but the IL-5 receptor seems to be shed from eosinophils found in BAL fluid, suggesting that eosinophils may become less responsive to IL-5 over time/with maturation.[16,17] Because IL-5 is believed to be produced primarily by lymphocytes, evaluating IL-5 protein in tissue is difficult. IL-5 messenger RNA (mRNA) is increased in bronchial biopsies of asthmatic patients, and has been suggested to correlate with disease severity.[18,19] Although early studies of all-comer asthmatics not subgrouped by eosinophilia were negative, 3 studies have recently been published that confirm the importance of IL-5 to asthmatic exacerbations, but only in a subgroup with blood or sputum eosinophilia.[20–24] In one of those studies, although the impact on blood eosinophils was profound, the effect on tissue (and sputum) eosinophils was less dramatic.[22]

Another factor closely linked to tissue eosinophils is the family of eosinophilic chemokines known as eotaxins. There are 3 identified eotaxins (1, 2, and 3), which do not share a similar structure but which all activate the CCR3 receptor present primarily on eosinophils. In contrast to IL-5, eotaxins are produced by structural cells, such as fibroblasts and epithelial cells, making eotaxins ideal candidate biomarkers to identify tissue (as opposed to luminal) eosinophils. Eotaxin promotes eosinophil tissue migration and has been shown to be increased both at the mRNA and protein level in the bronchial mucosa in asthmatics compared with nonasthmatic individuals.[25,26] Eotaxins are known to be strongly upregulated by Th2 cytokines, such as IL-4 and IL-13, which have also been linked to asthma.[27,28] Studies have shown Th2 cytokines IL-4 and IL-5 are increased in BAL fluid.[29] After segmental allergen challenge, IL-4 remained increased for at least 2 weeks and had a dose-dependent effect on α-smooth muscle actin and collagen III synthesis by human lung fibroblasts.[30]

Cysteinyl leukotrienes have also been found to be increased in BAL, urine, sputum, and exhaled breath condensate in asthmatic patients.[31–34] They act through the cysteinyl leukotriene 1 receptor, primarily, although LTE4 may preferentially activate a different receptor, the P2Y2 receptor, potentially explaining the increased tissue eosinophils seen after LTE4 inhalation.[35,36] Montelukast and zafirlukast are leukotriene receptor antagonists that selectively block the cysteinyl leukotriene 1 receptor.[37] These medications have been shown to decrease blood, sputum, and BAL eosinophils.[38,39] Moreover, the use of leukotriene receptor antagonists also decreased blood eosinophils in the pediatric population.[40]

Although its role in eosinophilic inflammation and asthma remains unclear, the eicosanoid 15-hyroxyeicosetetrenoic acid (15-HETE) and its enzyme, 15-lipoxygenase (LO), have also been reported to be increased in asthma, and particularly in severe eosinophilic asthma in both BAL and tissue (**Fig. 1**).[41] 15-HETE is also increased in wheezing children. 15-LO is upregulated by IL-4 and IL-13 in various cell types.[42,43] Clinical relevance for this increase in 15-LO1 is suggested by the observations that 15-LO and its product are critical for the generation of MUC5AC, a mucin believed to be of key importance to asthma.[44,45]

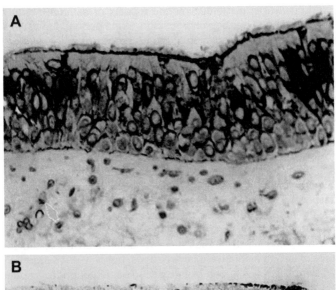

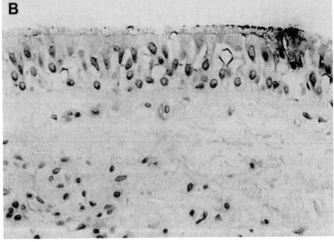

Fig. 1. Representative photomicrographs of 15-LO immunostaining in an eosinophil-positive severe asthmatic (*A*) and a normal individual. (*B*) Bronchial epithelial cells and inflammatory cells in the submucosa were stained for 15-LO (15-LO immunostaining, original magnification x400). (*From* Chu HW, Balzar S, Westcott JY, et al. Expression and activation of 15-lipoxygenase pathway in severe asthma: relationship to eosinophilic phenotype and collagen deposition. Clin Exp Allergy 2002;32:1561; with permission.)

BIOMARKERS FOR NEUTROPHILIC ASTHMA

Although numerous candidate tissue biomarkers have been identified for the eosinophilic phenotype of asthma, biomarkers for noneosinophilic asthma are not so well understood (see **Table 1**). Noneosinophilic asthma has been proposed to consist of 2 different subtypes: neutrophilic and paucigranulocytic,[46] and generally fall under the category of Th2-Lo asthma.[47] Of these subtypes, neutrophilic asthma has been associated with a more severe phenotype of asthma.[48,49] Sputum analysis of neutrophils more consistently discriminates severe asthma from milder asthma than tissue eosinophils. Sputum can also be followed serially over time. This neutrophilic type of asthma has been described in relation to increases in several proneutrophilic factors, including LTB4 and IL-8. LTB4 is a lipid mediator produced from arachidonic acid by the 5-LO enzyme. LTB4 has been noted to be increased in BAL fluid in relation to neutrophils in severe asthma, as well as in less severe patients with nocturnal asthma, LTB4 was also associated with eosinophilic inflammation.[50] Higher levels of LTB4 are also found in wheezing children defined as those with 2 episodes of wheezing or wheezing greater than or equal to 2 months in a 6-month period.[51] IL-8 is a potent neutrophilic chemokine produced by a variety of cell types, which in addition to being associated with neutrophilic asthma, has been suggested to increase with increasing severity of disease.[49] IL-8 in BAL fluid was significantly higher than serum and also higher in patients with asthma compared with patients with chronic obstructive pulmonary disease.[52] In contrast, in children, IL-8 levels in BAL were found to be similar to normal controls.[53]

Increased tissue and BAL neutrophils have also been linked to increases in matrix metalloproteinase-9 (MMP-9) in tissue and BAL fluid.[54,55] MMP-9 has been shown to be increased in the BAL in both adult and pediatric asthmatic patients.[56–58] MMP-9 exists in many forms, but needs to be activated before its gelatinolytic enzymatic properties are present. In most studies, most MMP-9 is in the inactive or pro form.[59] However, in severe asthma, there is an increase in the high-molecular-weight form of MMP-9, which is present when the MMP-9 is linked to a neutrophilic protein. This high-molecular-weight form is also less likely to be inhibited by inhibitors of MMPs.[59] Submucosal expression of MMP-9 has been reported to correlate with subepithelial thickness of the subepithelial basement membrane (SBM), as measured by collagen III expression, suggesting it may contribute in airway remodeling.[60] In addition, MMP-9 has been shown to be present within the subbasement membrane and to correlate with the level of neutrophils in the tissue, and the numbers of cells expressing transforming growth factor β (TGF-β). Both neutrophils and MMP-9 levels are also correlated with worsening forced expiratory volume in 1 second.[49,54]

Neutrophilic inflammation has also been proposed to be associated with activation of Th17 pathways. However, the tissue data to support this proposition in humans are still modest, including studies that suggest no relationship of IL-17 with neutrophilic inflammation.[61,62]

BIOMARKERS FOR PAUCIGRANULOCYTIC ASTHMA

Not all asthmatic patients have measurable eosinophilic or neutrophilic inflammation in tissue or BAL fluid (see **Table 1**). The mechanisms by which asthma exists in individuals with paucigranulocytic asthma are not clear; however, several possible explanations may exist. First, the patient may have undergone a degree of remodeling in their airways such that inflammation is no longer the primary cause for their disease. These patients may have more persistent airflow limitation and less variability in their disease.[4] Specific or reproducible biomarkers of remodeling in tissue are not yet available. It has been suggested that the amount of smooth muscle present in the tissue and the size of the smooth muscle cells are increased with increasing severity of asthma, and that these changes exist independent of inflammation.[63] However, these studies have not been replicated. Another group has reported mast cells to be increased in bronchial smooth muscle bundles and that this increase is specific to asthma.[64]

Because tissue inflammation is traditionally measured in proximal airways, as opposed to the distal lung, it is also possible that distal lung inflammation exists and persists in patients with little tissue inflammation in the proximal lung. Few studies have used distal lung tissue. However, mast cells, particularly chymase-positive mast cells, are increased in the distal lung in patients with severe asthma and correlate positively with lung function, suggesting that they may be protective in severe asthma.[65] The chymase-positive mast cell has also been shown to be increased in asthmatics and associated with increase in vessels and vascular endothelial growth factor expression.[66]

BIOMARKERS FOR REMODELING

Perhaps the greatest attention has been paid to the thickness of the SBM (see **Table 1**). Although it is clear that the SBM is a reasonable biomarker for asthma, the data to suggest that it is a biomarker for severity are less clear.[2,67–69] In addition, the thickness of the SBM has been reported to be higher in those with active eosinophilic inflammation as opposed to those with no or minimal eosinophilic inflammation.[2] The SBM is made up of a variety of different collagens (primarily I, III, and V), and numerous other extracellular matrix glycoproteins, including tenascin, lumican, decorin, and others. Tenascin expression was shown to be increased 24 hours after allergen inhalation challenge, returning to baseline levels at 7 days. In contrast, procollagen I and procollagen III expression was increased at 7 days after challenge.[70] Although the mechanisms for the increase in airway smooth muscle and SBM in asthma remain poorly understood, TGF-β has been suggested in several studies to play a critical role.[2,3,71,72] Increases in TGF-β can induce fibroblast proliferation and collagen synthesis. In severe asthma, TGF-β2 in particular has been associated with increased fibrosis.[72,73] Anti–IL-5 was shown to decrease matrix deposition in the SBM, while decreasing the levels of TGF-β in the tissue likely through an effect on eosinophils.[74]

SUMMARY

Although there are as of yet no biomarkers in lavage or lung tissue of sufficient validity to diagnose and manage asthma in general, recent efforts to phenotype asthma are strongly linked with the evolution of biomarkers specific to that phenotype. Because of the difficulty in obtaining these bronchoscopic specimens, it is unlikely that any factor in these compartments will achieve sufficient reproducibility or predictive value over time to be widely accepted as a clinically useful biomarker. However, efforts to compare tissue and lavage biomarkers with other, less invasive measures of sputum, serum, or exhaled breath may lead to better support for these systems. Sputum eosinophils are perhaps the best example, with tissue and lavage eosinophils studied first, but validated as a biomarker of poor asthma control, asthma exacerbations, and steroid responsiveness in the less invasive sputum studies. Further evaluation and understanding of these biomarkers in relation to phenotype, genotype, and less invasive measures that can be repeated over time should greatly enhance the use of these bronchoscopic findings.

REFERENCES

1. Bousquet J, Chanez P, Lacoste JY, et al. Eosinophilic inflammation in asthma. N Engl J Med 1990;323(15):1033–9.
2. Wenzel SE, Schwartz LB, Langmack EL, et al. Evidence that severe asthma can be divided pathologically into two inflammatory subtypes with distinct physiologic and clinical characteristics. Am J Respir Crit Care Med 1999;160(3):1001–8.

3. Miranda C, Busacker A, Balzar S, et al. Distinguishing severe asthma phenotypes: role of age at onset and eosinophilic inflammation. J Allergy Clin Immunol 2004;113(1):101–8.

4. Haldar P, Pavord ID. Noneosinophilic asthma: a distinct clinical and pathologic phenotype. J Allergy Clin Immunol 2007;119(5):1043–52.

5. Lemière C, Ernst P, Olivenstein R, et al. Airway inflammation assessed by invasive and noninvasive means in severe asthma: eosinophilic and noneosinophilic phenotypes. J Allergy Clin Immunol 2006;118(5):1033–9.

6. Green RH, Brightling CE, McKenna S, et al. Asthma exacerbations and sputum eosinophil counts: a randomised controlled trial. Lancet 2002;360(9347): 1715–21.

7. Jayaram L, Pizzichini MM, Cook RJ, et al. Determining asthma treatment by monitoring sputum cell counts: effect on exacerbations. Eur Respir J 2006;27(3): 483–94.

8. Wenzel SE. Severe asthma in adults. Am J Respir Crit Care Med 2005;172(2): 149–60.

9. Silkoff PE, Lent AM, Busacker AA, et al. Exhaled nitric oxide identifies the persistent eosinophilic phenotype in severe refractory asthma. J Allergy Clin Immunol 2005;116(6):1249–55.

10. Menzies-Gow A, Flood-Page P, Sehmi R, et al. Anti-IL-5 (mepolizumab) therapy induces bone marrow eosinophil maturational arrest and decreases eosinophil progenitors in the bronchial mucosa of atopic asthmatics. J Allergy Clin Immunol 2003;111(4):714–9.

11. Yamaguchi Y, Suda T, Suda J, et al. Purified interleukin 5 supports the terminal differentiation and proliferation of murine eosinophilic precursors. J Exp Med 1988;167(1):43–56.

12. Palframan RT, Collins PD, Severs NJ, et al. Mechanisms of acute eosinophil mobilization from the bone marrow stimulated by interleukin 5: the role of specific adhesion molecules and phosphatidylinositol 3-kinase. J Exp Med 1998;188(9): 1621–32.

13. Tavernier J, Van de Heyen J, Verhee A, et al. Interleukin-5 regulates the isoform expression of its own receptor alpha-subunit. Blood 2000;95(5):1600–7.

14. Sehmi R, Wood LJ, Watson R, et al. Allergen-induced increases in IL-5 receptor alpha-subunit expression on bone marrow-derived CD34+cells from asthmatic subjects. A novel marker of progenitor cell commitment towards eosinophilic differentiation. J Clin Invest 1997;100(10):2466–75.

15. Menzies-Gow AN, Flood-Page PT, Robinson DS, et al. Effect of inhaled interleukin-5 on eosinophil progenitors in the bronchi and bone marrow of asthmatics and non-asthmatic volunteers. Clin Exp Allergy 2007;37(7):1023–32.

16. Kelly EA, Rodriguez RR, Busse WW, et al. The effect of segmental bronchoprovocation with allergen on airway lymphocyte function. Am J Respir Crit Care Med 1997;156(5):1421–8.

17. Liu LY, Sedgwick JB, Bates ME, et al. Decreased expression of membrane IL-5 receptor alpha on human eosinophils: I. Loss of membrane IL-5 receptor alpha on airway eosinophils and increased soluble IL-5 receptor alpha in the airway after allergen challenge. J Immunol 2002;169(11):6452–8.

18. Hamid Q, Azzawi M, Ying S, et al. Expression of mRNA for IL-5 in mucosal bronchial biopsies from asthma. J Clin Invest 1991;87(5):1541–6.

19. Humbert M, Corrigan CJ, Kimmitt P, et al. Relationship between IL-4 and IL-5 mRNA expression and disease severity in atopic asthma. Am J Respir Crit Care Med 1997;156(3 Pt 1):704–8.

20. Flood-Page P, Swenson C, Faiferman I, et al, International Mepolizumab Study Group. A study to evaluate safety and efficacy of mepolizumab in patients with moderate persistent asthma. Am J Respir Crit Care Med 2007;176(11):1062–71 [Epub 2007 Sep 13. PubMed PMID: 17872493].

21. Leckie MJ, ten Brinke A, Khan J, et al. Effects of an interleukin-5 blocking monoclonal antibody on eosinophils, airway hyper-responsiveness, and the late asthmatic response. Lancet 2000;356(9248):2144–8.

22. Haldar P, Brightling CE, Hargadon B, et al. Mepolizumab and exacerbations of refractory eosinophilic asthma. N Engl J Med 2009;360(10):973–84 [Erratum in: N Engl J Med. 2011 Feb 10;364(6):588. PubMed PMID: 19264686].

23. Castro M, Mathur S, Hargreave F, et al, Res-5-0010 Study Group. Reslizumab for poorly controlled, eosinophilic asthma: a randomized, placebo-controlled study. Am J Respir Crit Care Med 2011;184(10):1125–32 [Epub 2011 Aug 18. PubMed PMID: 21852542].

24. Nair P, Pizzichini MM, Kjarsgaard M, et al. Mepolizumab for prednisone-dependent asthma with sputum eosinophilia. N Engl J Med 2009;360(10):985–93 [PubMed PMID: 19264687].

25. Lamkhioued B, Renzi PM, Abi-Younes S, et al. Increased expression of eotaxin in bronchoalveolar lavage and airways of asthmatics contributes to the chemotaxis of eosinophils to the site of inflammation. J Immunol 1997;159(9):4593–601.

26. Ying S, Robinson DS, Meng Q, et al. Enhanced expression of eotaxin and CCR3 mRNA and protein in atopic asthma: association with airway hyperresponsiveness and predominant co-localization of eotaxin in mRNA to bronchial epithelial and endothelial cells. Eur J Immunol 1997;27(12):3507–16.

27. Lamkhioued B, Abddelilah SG, Hamid Q, et al. The CCR3 receptor is involved in eosinophil differentiation and is up-regulated by Th2 cytokines in CD34+ progenitor cells. J Immunol 2003;170(1):537–47.

28. Li L, Xia Y, Nguyen A, et al. Effects of Th2 cytokines on chemokine expression in the lung: IL-13 potently induces eotaxin expression by airway epithelial cells. J Immunol 1999;162(5):2477–87.

29. Adelroth E. How to measure airway inflammation: bronchoalveolar lavage and airway biopsies. Can Respir J 1998;5(Suppl A):18A–21A.

30. Batra V, Musani AI, Hastie AT, et al. Bronchoalveolar lavage fluid concentrations of transforming growth factor (TGF)-beta1, TGF-beta2, interleukin (IL)-4 and IL-13 after segmental allergen challenge and their effects on alpha-smooth muscle actin and collagen III synthesis by primary human lung fibroblasts. Clin Exp Allergy 2004;34(3):437–44.

31. Wenzel SE, Larsen GL, Johnston K, et al. Elevated levels of leukotriene C4 in bronchoalveolar lavage fluid from atopic asthmatics after endobronchial allergen challenge. Am Rev Respir Dis 1990;142(1):112–9.

32. Taylor GW, Taylor I, Black P, et al. Urinary leukotriene E4 after antigen challenge and in acute asthma and allergic rhinitis. Lancet 1989;1(8638):584–8.

33. Pavord ID, Ward R, Woltmann G, et al. Induced sputum eicosanoid concentrations in asthma. Am J Respir Crit Care Med 1999;160(6):1905–9.

34. Montuschi P, Barnes PJ. Exhaled leukotrienes and prostaglandins in asthma. J Allergy Clin Immunol 2002;109(4):615–20.

35. Laitinen A, Lindqvist A, Halme M, et al. Leukotriene E(4)-induced persistent eosinophilia and airway obstruction are reversed by zafirlukast in patients with asthma. J Allergy Clin Immunol 2005;115(2):259–65 [PubMed PMID: 15696079].

36. Laitinen LA, Laitinen A, Haahtela T, et al. Leukotriene E4 and granulocytic infiltration into asthmatic airways. Lancet 1993;341(8851):989–90 [PubMed PMID: 8096945].
37. Lynch KR, O'Neill GP, Liu Q, et al. Characterization of the human cysteinyl leukotriene CysLT1 receptor. Nature 1999;399(6738):789–93.
38. Pizzichini E, Le JA, Reiss TF, et al. Montelukast reduces airway eosinophilic inflammation in asthma: a randomized, controlled trial. Eur Respir J 1999;14(1):12–8.
39. Calhoun WJ, Lavins BJ, Minkwitz MC, et al. Effect of zafirlukast (Accolate) on cellular mediators of inflammation: bronchoalveolar lavage fluid findings after segmental antigen challenge. Am J Respir Crit Care Med 1998;157(5 Pt 1): 1381–9.
40. Stelmach I, Jerzynska J, Kunan P. A randomized, double-blind trial of the effect of treatment with montelukast on bronchial hyperresponsiveness and serum eosinophilic cationic protein (ECP), soluble interleukin 2 receptor (sIL-2R), IL-4, and soluble intercellular adhesion molecule 1 (sICAM-1) in children with asthma. J Allergy Clin Immunol 2002;109(2):257–63.
41. Chu HW, Balzar S, Westcott JY, et al. Expression and activation of 15-lipoxygenase pathway in severe asthma: relationship to eosinophilic phenotype and collagen deposition. Clin Exp Allergy 2002;32(11):1558–65.
42. Nassar GM, Morrow JD, Roberts LJ II, et al. Induction of 15-lipoxygenase by interleukin 13 in human blood monocytes. J Biol Chem 1994;269(44):27631–4.
43. Profita M, Vignola AM, Sala A, et al. Interleukin-4 enhances 15-lipoxygenase activity and incorporation of 15(S)-HETE into cellular phospholipids in cultured pulmonary epithelial cells. Am J Respir Cell Mol Biol 1999;20(1):61–8.
44. Zhao J, O'Donnell VB, Balzar S, et al. 15-Lipoxygenase 1 interacts with phosphatidylethanolamine-binding protein to regulate MAPK signaling in human airway epithelial cells. Proc Natl Acad Sci U S A 2011;108(34):14246–51 [Epub 2011 Aug 9. PubMed PMID: 21831839; PubMed Central PMCID: PMC3161579].
45. Zhao J, Maskrey B, Balzar S, et al. Interleukin-13-induced MUC5AC is regulated by 15-lipoxygenase 1 pathway in human bronchial epithelial cells. Am J Respir Crit Care Med 2009;179(9):782–90 [Epub 2009 Feb 12. PubMed PMID: 19218191; PubMed Central PMCID: PMC2675565].
46. Douwes J, Gibson P, Pekkanen J, et al. Non-eosinophilic asthma: importance and possible mechanisms. Thorax 2002;57(7):643–8.
47. Wenzel SE. Asthma phenotypes: the evolution from clinical to molecular approaches. Nat Med 2012;18(5):716–25. http://dx.doi.org/10.1038/nm, 2678. PubMed PMID: 22561835.
48. Wenzel SE, Szefler SJ, Leung DY, et al. Bronchoscopic evaluation of severe asthma: persistent inflammation associated with high dose glucocorticoids. Am J Respir Crit Care Med 1997;156(3 Pt 1):737–43.
49. Jatakanon A, Uasuf C, Maziak W, et al. Neutrophilic inflammation in severe persistent asthma. Am J Respir Crit Care Med 1999;160(5 Pt 1):1532–9.
50. Wenzel SE, Trudeau JB, Kaminsky DA, et al. Effect of 5-lipoxygenase inhibition on bronchoconstriction and airway inflammation in nocturnal asthma. Am J Respir Crit Care Med 1995;152(3):897–905.
51. Krawiec ME, Westcott JY, Chu HW, et al. Persistent wheezing in very young children is associated with lower respiratory inflammation. Am J Respir Crit Care Med 2001;163(6):1338–43.
52. Hollander C, Sitkauskiene B, Sakalauskas R, et al. Serum and bronchial lavage fluid concentrations of IL-8 SLPI, sCD14, and sICAM-1 in patients with COPD and asthma. Respir Med 2007;101(9):1947–53.

53. Kim CK, Kim SW, Kim YK, et al. Bronchoalveolar lavage eosinophil cationic protein and interleukin-8 levels in acute asthma and acute bronchiolitis. Clin Exp Allergy 2005;35(5):591–7.

54. Wenzel SE, Balzar S, Cundall M, et al. Subepithelial basement membrane immunoreactivity for matrix metalloproteinase 9: association with asthma severity, neutrophilic inflammation, and wound repair. J Allergy Clin Immunol 2003; 111(6):1345–52.

55. Ohbayashi H, Shimokata K. Matrix metalloproteinase-9 and airway remodeling in asthma. Curr Drug Targets Inflamm Allergy 2005;4(2):177–81.

56. Mautino G, Oliver N, Chanez P, et al. Increased release of matrix matelloproteinase-9 in bronchoalveolar lavage fluid and by alveolar macrophages of asthmatics. Am J Respir Cell Mol Biol 1997;17(5):583–91.

57. Ko FW, Diba C, Roth M, et al. A comparison of airway and serum matrix metalloproteinase-9 activity among normal subjects, asthmatic patients, and patients with asthmatic mucus hypersecretion. Chest 2005;127(6):1919–27.

58. Tang LF, Du LZ, Chen ZM, et al. Levels of matrix metalloproteinase-9 and its inhibitor in bronchoalveolar lavage cells of asthmatic children. Fetal Pediatr Pathol 2006;25(1):1–7.

59. Cundall M, Sun Y, Miranda C, et al. Neutrophil-derived matrix metalloproteinase-9 is increased in severe asthma and poorly inhibited by glucocorticoids. J Allergy Clin Immunol 2003;112(6):1064–71.

60. Hoshino M, Nakamura Y, Sim J, et al. Bronchial subepithelial fibrosis and expression of matrix metalloproteinase-9 in asthmatic airway inflammation. J Allergy Clin Immunol 1998;102(5):783–8.

61. Chakir J, Shannon J, Molet S, et al. Airway remodeling-associated mediators in moderate to severe asthma: effect of steroids on TGF-beta, IL-11, IL-17, and type I and type III collagen expression. J Allergy Clin Immunol 2003;111(6): 1293–8 [PubMed PMID: 12789232].

62. Doe C, Bafadhel M, Siddiqui S, et al. Expression of the T helper 17-associated cytokines IL-17A and IL-17F in asthma and COPD. Chest 2010;138(5):1140–7 [Epub 2010 Jun 10. PubMed PMID: 20538817; PubMed Central PMCID: PMC2972626].

63. Benayoun L, Druilhe A, Dombret MC, et al. Airway structural alterations selectively associated with severe asthma. Am J Respir Crit Care Med 2003;167(10): 1360–8.

64. Brightling CE, Bradding P, Symon FA, et al. Mast-cell infiltration of airway smooth muscle in asthma. N Engl J Med 2002;346(22):1699–705 PMID: 12037149.

65. Balzar S, Chu HW, Strand M, et al. Relationship of small airway chymase-positive mast cells and lung function in severe asthma. Am J Respir Crit Care Med 2005; 171(5):431–9.

66. Zanini A, Chetta A, Saetta M, et al. Chymase-positive mast cells play a role in the vascular component of airway remodeling in asthma. J Allergy Clin Immunol 2007;120(2):329–33.

67. Chetta A, Foresi A, Del Donno M, et al. Airways remodeling is a distinctive feature of asthma and is related to severity of disease. Chest 1997;111(4):852–7.

68. Chu HW, Halliday JL, Martin RJ, et al. Collagen deposition in large airways may not differentiate severe asthma from milder forms of the disease. Am J Respir Crit Care Med 1998;158(6):1936–44.

69. Bourdin A, Neveu D, Vachier I, et al. Specificity of basement membrane thickening in severe asthma. J Allergy Clin Immunol 2007;119(6):1367–74.

70. Kariyawasam HH, Aizen M, Barkans J, et al. Remodeling and airway hyperresponsiveness but not cellular inflammation persists after allergen challenge in asthma. Am J Respir Crit Care Med 2007;175(9):896–904.
71. Minshall EM, Leung DY, Martin RJ, et al. Eosinophil-associated TGF-beta1 mRNA expression and airways fibrosis in bronchial asthma. Am J Respir Cell Mol Biol 1997;17(3):326–33.
72. Balzar S, Chu H, Silko P, et al. Increased TGF-beta2 in severe asthma with eosinophilia. J Allergy Clin Immunol 2005;115(1):110–7.
73. Chu HW, Trudeau JB, Balzar S, et al. Peripheral blood and airway tissue expression of transforming growth factor beta by neutrophils in asthmatic subjects and normal control subjects. J Allergy Clin Immunol 2000;106(6):1115–23.
74. Flood-Page P, Menzies-Gow A, Phipps S, et al. Anti-IL-5 treatment reduces deposition of ECM proteins in the bronchial subepithelial basement membrane of mild atopic asthmatics. J Clin Invest 2003;112(7):1029–36.

Bronchoprovocation Testing in Asthma

Rohit K. Katial, MD[a],*, Ronina A. Covar, MD[b]

KEYWORDS

- Bronchoprovocation testing • Asthma • Bronchial hyper-responsivenes
- Bronchoprovocation challenges

KEY POINTS

- Bronchial hyper-responsiveness (BHR) probably represents several inherent elements of the disease process, such as genetic predisposition, airway inflammation, and airway remodeling.
- Airway inflammation seems to account for the transient and variable component of BHR.
- The permanent or persistent component of BHR, particularly to direct stimuli, correlates significantly with structural changes in the airway, such as basement membrane thickness and epithelial damage.
- Trials of specific immunomodulatory therapy have shown considerable improvements in markers of airway inflammation, without significantly modifying airway reactivity.

Bronchial hyperresponsiveness (BHR) is defined as a heightened bronchoconstrictive response to airway stimuli. It complements the key features in asthma, such as variable or reversible airflow limitation and airway inflammation. To what extent the mechanisms of airflow limitation, airway inflammation, and BHR overlap is still unclear, and how these 3 components come together probably accounts for the wide variability of asthma as a disease. Although this property of the airway is dynamic, it can vary over time, with disease activity, triggers or specific exposure, and with treatment, there is a component that is not reflective of a specific disease entity. BHR has been documented in asymptomatic subjects in the general population and in other diseases as such as chronic obstructive pulmonary diseases, congestive heart failure, cystic.fibrosis, bronchitis, allergic rhinitis, and even in healthy subjects.[1–4] Whether its presence in these conditions indicates a common inflammatory process is still poorly understood.

Bronchoprovocation challenges (BPCs), using pharmacologic or physical means to evaluate BHR, have been used to serve a variety of purposes. The most common application of BPC is when a diagnosis of asthma in either a clinical or research

[a] Department of Medicine, National Jewish Health, 1400 Jackson Street (J329), Denver, CO 80206, USA; [b] Department of Pediatrics, National Jewish Health, 1400 Jackson Street (J316), Denver, CO 80206, USA
* Corresponding author.
E-mail address: KatialR@njhealth.org

Immunol Allergy Clin N Am 32 (2012) 413–431
http://dx.doi.org/10.1016/j.iac.2012.06.002
0889-8561/12/$ – see front matter © 2012 Elsevier Inc. All rights reserved.

(clinical trials and epidemiologic) setting is in question (eg, in patients who have symptoms but no other objective features of asthma such as airflow limitation). In general, the reliability of the test is more useful in excluding a diagnosis than in confirming one, based on the higher negative predictive value compared with its positive predictive ability.[5] This is more relevant in special situations, such as involvement in high-risk occupational tasks and environmental exposure (eg, military, scuba diving); however, because of the overlap in provocation doses causing a reduction in lung function at the time of a challenge between diseased and healthy subjects, setting an absolute level to define a diseased state is difficult.[6]

BPC can also be considered for patients who are suspected of having poor symptom perception, or for detecting peculiar physiologic features characteristic of certain asthmatics, such as presence of 'excessive' airway closure (characterized by lack of plateau on the dose–response curve)[7] BPCs have also become an important research outcome measure to monitor intervention outcome and determine mechanisms underlying efficacy. The use of BPC compared with clinical practice guidelines as a strategic tool to aid in the titration of inhaled corticosteroid dosing has been found to be effective at improving not only clinical parameters of asthma control, but also at alleviating airway inflammation.[8] BHR is related to various measures of asthma severity,[3,9,10] and it has also been reported as a predictor of development of persistent asthma[11,12] and airflow limitation in adulthood.[13] These significant applications of BPCs make them a requirement, and in many instances the gold standard, in the evaluation of asthma. Hence, it is important to reflect on what these tests convey about asthma.

Central to the application and interpretation of BPCs is understanding and standardizing the numerous BPCs available. This article covers the relationships between BHR and airway inflammation. Recent evidence suggests strongly that indeed, various commonly used BPCs differ in their potential to serve as inflammatory biomarkers: direct (eg, methacholine and histamine) and indirect (eg, exercise, adenosine, hypertonic saline, and mannitol). The response to direct stimuli is dependent on the smooth muscle's response to the chemical, whereas in indirect challenges, the reaction is caused by the smooth muscle's responsiveness to the mediators induced by the stimuli. The information obtained from numerous studies with BPC has provided valuable insights into the pathogenesis and pathophysiology of asthma, and the relationships between airway inflammation and BHR.

WHAT FACTORS CONSTITUTE BHR?
Genetic Component

There is evidence of genetic susceptibility not only to asthma and atopy, but more specifically to BHR, from clustering of these conditions in families.[14] For instance, the association of asthma, atopy, and BHR was stronger between identical twins compared with dizygotic twins. The strong correlations in monozygotic twins suggest an overlap between these genetic factors involved in each of these traits.[15] Coinheritance and colocalization of a gene to a region of chromosome 5q31–q33 that determines both BHR to histamine and serum immunoglobulin E (IgE) levels have been reported.[16] In that study, elevated levels of serum IgE were coinherited in siblings with BHR, but BHR was not correlated in siblings concordant for elevated serum IgE. These findings suggest that different genetic and environmental factors influence serum IgE levels, not necessarily affecting BHR. There are also several airway inflammatory mediators that are linked to chromosome 5q31–q33, such as granulocyte macrophage colony stimulating factor (GMCSF), fibroblast growth factor acidic, other colony-stimulating factors and receptors, the lymphocyte-specific glucocorticoid receptor 1, beta2-adrenergic receptor, and interleukin (IL)-3, IL-4, IL-5, IL9 and IL-13.[16] Colocalization of these genes in that region may account for the common pathophysiologic features of asthma involving IL-4 in isotype switch to IgE, and IL-3, IL-5, and GMCSF for proliferation and activation of eosinophils.

There are other genetic studies that link atopy or serum IgE levels or asthma to BHR, located in other regions such as in chromosome 11[17] and in the IL-4 and IL-13 cytokine region of chromosome 5,[18] more proximal to that found by Postma and colleagues.[16]

These findings still await confirmation in other populations, and no definite gene has been identified to date to account for BHR. In addition, recent evidence that gene–environment interaction such as with exposure to early environmental factors such as passive smoke (or other factors related to tobacco smoke in early life, such as viral infections) may modulate the genetic susceptibility for asthma-related phenotype.[19,20]

Transient and Permanent Components of BHR

In asthma, BHR can be variable both within and between individuals. The variability emanates from different etiology in addition to genetic predisposition: presence of structural changes that account for more permanent component and the degree or severity of airway inflammation that contributes to the transient or modifiable elements. O'Byrne and Inman[21] proposed the terms persistent and transient, respectively, to differentiate these elements. For example, recent exposures to allergen,[22–25] ozone,[26] infection,[27,28] or occupational triggers[29,30] contribute to the transient property, whereas structural changes impact the permanent or persistent component.

The role of airway smooth muscle in bronchoconstriction and BHR is well recognized, but whether there are unique inherent airway smooth muscle characteristics or whether airway smooth muscle is merely an effector of an abnormal inflammatory response is unclear. Airway inflammation is critical in the pathogenesis of asthma. What specific component of the inflammatory cascade and to what extent inflammation impacts BHR are disputed. Furthermore, the physiologic and structural changes characteristic of airway remodeling (ie, fibrosis, airway smooth muscle hypertrophy, extracellular matrix deposition, vascularity) or epithelial damage[31] probably have a greater impact over airway inflammation on the more permanent feature of BHR.[32] In a double-blind, randomized, placebo-controlled, parallel group study, the relationships between airflow limitation, airway inflammation, airway remodeling, and BHR before and after treatment with high-dose inhaled flucatisone propionate (FP 750 µg twice daily) were evaluated in a group of patients who had mild persistent asthma.[33] Multiple regression analysis indicated that the 40% of the variability in BHR consisted of 21% being related to reticular basement membrane thickness ($P = .009$), 11% to bronchoalveolar lavage epithelial cells ($P = .04$), and 8% to bronchoalveolar lavage eosinophils ($P = .046$), with spirometric indices and mast cells being insignificant predictors of BHR. The longitudinal data validated the cross-sectional model. Spirometric indices and cellular inflammation improved after 3 months of treatment, with no further improvement at 12 months, whereas BHR improved throughout the 1-year study, represented by 6 doubling dose changes. A reduction in reticular basement membrane thickness serving as an index of airway remodeling was evident much later, only after 12 months of treatment (mean change 1.9, 95% confidence interval [CI] -3 to 0.7 µm; $P = .01$ vs baseline, $P = .05$ vs placebo). Early changes in BHR (ie, 2 doubling dose magnitude) could be accounted for by improvement in airway inflammation within 3 months, and subsequent improvement by airway remodeling.[33] Hence, both airway inflammation and airway remodeling contribute to BHR, and this study provides cross-sectional and longitudinal support that a larger contribution comes from features of airway remodeling. Both features of airway inflammation and remodeling respond, albeit temporally different, to anti-inflammatory treatment.

What makes the issue more complex is that the actual method of bronchoprovocation may provide a diverse relationship between inflammation and BHR. Indirect challenges are presumed to be more reflective of airway inflammation, in contrast to direct stimuli, which are more related to the irreversible or persistent BHR. It is likely that there are many variables contributing to BHR and in specific conditions, different mechanisms or a combination thereof are responsible.

The Link Between BHR and Airway Inflammation

Associations between BHR and other inflammatory biomarkers

Evidence in support of this relationship can be grouped according to associations between inflammatory and allergic markers and BHR, and modification of BHR and inflammatory markers using anti-inflammatory medications.

Sensitization and allergen challenge or exposure in animal and human studies using single or repeated doses induces airway reactivity that is associated with a variety of immunologic features, such as production of antigen specific IgE levels, up-regulation of T-helper cytokines, early and late-phase reactions, and eosinophilic inflammation.[34–37] After allergen stimulation, the influx of inflammatory cells in the airways, notably eosinophils, precedes the development of late-phase response, and correlates with an increase in BHR. The onslaught of inflammatory cells in the airways at the time of the allergen challenge suggests a causal relationship between BHR and airway inflammation. Whether the effect is caused by activation of eosinophils releasing substances that can increase reactivity, or produced by the epithelial damage itself, which enhances BHR, is not well established.

Associations between BHR and other inflammatory processes or markers not necessarily characteristic of purely eosinophilic process exist. Using a murine model for asthma, mice that had been sensitized with ovalbumin and then challenged repeatedly with ovalbumin aerosols were treated with monoclonal antibodies directed against IL-4, IL-5, interferon (IFN)-g, or tumor necrosis factor (TNF)-a during the challenge period.[38] The control antibody-treated mice showed hyper-responsiveness to methacholine and presence of eosinophils in bronchoalveolar lavage. Treatment with antibodies to IL-4 or IL-5 did not inhibit BHR, although IL-5 specifically inhibited bronchoalveolar lavage eosinophilia in ovalbumin-challenged mice. In contrast, IFN-g completely abolished, and TNF-a partially but not significantly inhibited development of airway hyper-responsiveness in ovalbumin-challenged animals, with neither treatment having an effect on eosinophilia.[38]

In another murine model, the ability to develop BHR also did not correlate with the degree of airway eosinophilia, inflammation, or total serum and OVA-specific IgE levels in genetically different inbred mouse strains (BALB/c, B6D2F1, and C57BL/6).[39] Higher BHR was found in the BALB strain that was associated with lower levels of eosinophils and OVA-specific IgE levels, compared with the B6D2F1 strain. Hence, there is an apparent dissociation between eosinophilia and antigen-specific IgE and BHR. In addition, the genetic background of the mice influenced the development of BHR.

These observations, specifically that of inhibition of BHR using specific mediators exclusive of an effect on airway eosinophilia, and the dissociation between airway eosinophilia and BHR, suggest that other mechanisms are involved. T lymphocytes have been shown to play a role in both intrinsic, nonatopic BHR and the development of antigen-induced BHR.[40–42] Alveolar macrophages may play a role in the development of nonspecific BHR, because these were the only cell types significantly increased in rats receiving repeated antigen challenges.[43] This is supported by a study in people in whom nonspecific BHR to histamine was closely correlated with elevated eosinophils and macrophages, and with the ratio of eosinophils to macrophages.[44] Airway mast cells and eosinophils were found to correlate with BHR in asthmatics treated with corticosteroids.[45] A study by Kelly and colleagues[46] also suggests a relation between bronchial responsiveness and both neutrophil numbers and macrophage activity.

Although still speculative, different immune profiles may be involved in the development of BHR based on atopy. Among nonatopics, elevated allergen-specific and polyclonal IL-10 production, TNF-a, and IFN-g were associated with BHR, whereas BHR among atopic individuals was associated with eosinophilia, IL-5, and IgE.[47]

There are numerous epidemiologic and clinical trial studies that present associations, albeit modest, between BHR and features of atopy or other biomarkers of eosinophilic inflammation in the airway (from sputum, bronchoalveolar lavage, and exhaled substances).[44,48–56] The associations with various measures of atopy can be variable. For example, in a study by Jansen and colleagues,[57] eosinophilia (odds ratio [OR] = 2.06, 95% CI, 1.28–3.31) and skin test positivity (OR = 1.66, 95% CI, 1.02–2.71) were both significantly associated with BHR to histamine, but high serum total IgE levels were not (OR = 1.29, 95% CI, 0.81–2.03) associated with BHR in this middle-aged population. In addition, the significant association between BHR and positive skin test pertained to symptomatic subjects only (OR = 5.78, 95% CI, 1.63–20.51), independent of eosinophilia and high serum total IgE levels. In contrast, the relationship between peripheral blood eosinophilia and BHR was the same in asymptomatic subjects and symptomatic subjects.[57] These findings suggest that skin testing, serum total IgE level, and peripheral blood eosinophilia represent different features of the atopic phenotype, with eosinophilia having the most robust association with BHR.

In the past decade, there has been a surge in the application of a noninvasive measure of airway inflammation in asthma using exhaled nitric oxide. This biomarker has been correlated with BHR both in corticosteroid naive and treated subjects.[45,58,59] With significant associations reported between exhaled nitric oxide levels and BHR, the feasibility of using exhaled nitric oxide measurements makes it a more attractive surrogate biomarker over BHR; however, the association is still quite modest (with approximately 9%–16% of exhaled nitric oxide variability probably attributable to BHR). Therefore, different mechanisms underlie exhaled nitric oxide measurements and BHR.

Although numerous studies illustrate the link between BHR and various measures of airway inflammation, there are studies that show a lack of an association.[31,60–65] Crimi and colleagues[65] evaluated the relationships between BHR and the number and types of inflammatory cells in the sputum, bronchoalveolar lavage, and bronchial biopsy samples of patients who had mild-to-moderate asthma with sensitization to either house dust mite or animal dander. In this study, no association was found between BHR and the presence of inflammatory cells (eosinophils, neutrophils, lymphocytes, or macrophages) in the airways. It could also be possible that it is not just the presence or number of inflammatory cells per se, but the activation of these cells that would correlate with BHR. Perhaps the correlation between role for eosinophils in allergic inflammation and BHR would be more apparent after an allergen challenge, and not necessarily at steady state or baseline.[66]

Modifying BHR Using Anti-inflammatory and Immunomodulatory Therapy

More than just associations of BHR with various surrogates of airway inflammation, convincing evidence supportive of the premise that BHR is indeed a biomarker of airway inflammation comes from numerous clinical trials demonstrating favorable effects of anti-inflammatory medications such as inhaled corticosteroids and leukotriene-modifying agents on BHR and other inflammatory indices.[33,67–70] Despite significantly improving symptoms and decreasing airway inflammation, inhaled corticosteroids produce at best a modest decrease in BHR as measured by histamine or methacholine challenges: a magnitude of 1.5 to 6 doubling dose reduction in BHR.[33,69,71,72] This suggests that the effect of treatment on BHR is not absolute, despite normalization of lung function or amelioration of symptoms and inflammation. In addition to inhaled corticosteroids, other interventions such as leukotriene inhibitor and receptor antagonists[73–76] and environmental interventions have been shown to reduce bronchial reactivity.[77,78]

In contrast to the interventions that target a broader influence on the inflammatory response, specific immunomodulation in human studies has afforded no significant effect on BHR, despite a substantial bearing on inflammatory markers. In a randomized, double-blind, parallel, placebo-controlled study in people who had allergic asthma,[79] single infusion of anti-IL-5 (either 2.5 mg/kg or 10 mg/kg) failed to modify BHR to histamine before and after allergen challenge 1 week and 1 month after the dose, despite a long-term decrease in peripheral blood and sputum eosinophils. These findings suggest that eosinophilia might not be the prime factor responsible for BHR in allergic asthma, because several inflammatory cells (eg, T cells, mast cells, eosinophils) contribute to the late asthmatic response, so that anti-inflammatory compounds that have broader coverage might be more effective at targeting this outcome. In addition, anti-IgE (omalizumab) treatment for 16 weeks given to adults who have mild-to-moderate asthma afforded a marked reduction in serum IgE, a reduction of IgE-þ cells in the airway mucosa, sputum eosinophil count, tissue eosinophils, cells positive for the high-affinity Fc receptor for IgE, CD3þ, CD4þ, and CD8þ T lymphocytes, B lymphocytes, and cells staining for iIL-4, without an effect on BHR to methacholine responsiveness.[80] These studies suggest that, at least in allergic asthma, specific therapy directed at eosinophil or IgE regulation does not obliterate bronchial responsiveness to methacholine.

Although the effects of certain immunomodulatory interventions on BHR are limited, BHR can still be used as a target for medication adjustment. The results of a study allowing titration of treatment with inhaled corticosteroid based on the degree of airway responsiveness to methacholine (BHR strategy) compared with standard clinical guidelines (reference strategy based solely on symptoms and lung function)[8] provide more indirect but strong evidence of BHR being a surrogate marker of inflammation in asthma. Participants whose treatment was adjusted based on their BHR had less exacerbation (0.23 and 0.43 exacerbation/year/patient, respectively) and greater improvement in lung function, but required higher doses of inhaled corticosteroids compared with subjects whose treatment was titrated according to recommended clinical guidelines. Of interest, bronchial biopsy findings showed greater reduction in thickness of the subepithelial reticular layer in the BHR strategy group than in the reference strategy group. The changes in BHR in both strategy groups were correlated with eosinophil counts in the biopsies ($r = -0.48$, $P = .003$).[8]

In summary, even if a general association exists between BHR and airway inflammation in asthma, such a relationship is not absolute and is therefore limited, because both measures can be influenced by different factors. It is likely that single measurements of BHR to pharmacologic stimuli cannot provide accurate information on airway inflammation. Depending on the BPC used, they could be suggestive of a different disease or immunologic pathway.

Correlations Between Direct and Indirect Challenges

The manner in which BPCs are conducted can be relevant in defining the association between BHR and airway inflammation; hence the distinction between direct and indirect stimuli is made. BPCs using direct stimuli such as methacholine and histamine provoke bronchoconstriction by acting primarily on airway smooth muscles and also on mucus glands and airway microvasculature. Methacholine (acetyl-b-methylcholine chloride), a synthetic derivative of acetylcholine, binds to specific muscarinic receptors, whereas histamine binds to H1 receptors on the airway smooth muscle. In contrast, indirect challenges use stimuli (eg, physical, osmotic, or pharmacologic) that affect inflammatory and neuronal cells, and induce release of mediators or cytokines that cause bronchospasm. Examples of stimuli acting indirectly to assess BHR include exercise, adenosine monophosphate (AMP), dry powder mannitol, and eucapnic voluntary hyperpnoea (EVH). This section presents correlations between direct and indirect BPC and compares the effects of anti-inflammatory therapy in regard to symptoms, markers of airway inflammation, and BHR using direct and indirect airway challenges.

The most common pharmacologic agents used for direct challenges are methacholine and histamine; their pharmacokinetic properties are known, and their safety has long been established. Bronchial responsiveness to methacholine and histamine correlates significantly (r = 0.9).[81] BPCs using histamine and methacholine are considered to be sensitive in diagnosing asthma, particularly in patients who have asthma symptoms. Because of the continuous variable using PC20 and the overlap in PC20 results between healthy and diseased patients, a careful decision analysis taking into consideration pretest probability and post-test probability is recommended when interpreting the results (**Fig. 1**).[4]

The pretest probability is an estimate of the likelihood of asthma before the procedure is obtained. The post-test probability is the likelihood of asthma taking into account the pretest probability and the methacholine provocation results, so that the actual PC20 results represent the contribution of the BPC to the diagnosis. For example, in an epidemiologic survey of asthma with a randomly selected sample whose medical history is not as detailed, an estimate of prevalence or pretest probability would be 5%. Subjects who would have a PC20 of 1 mg/mL could have an approximate 45% post-test

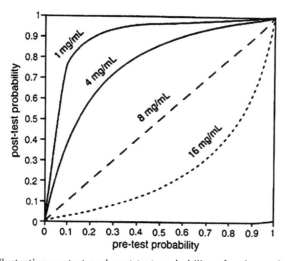

Fig. 1. Curves illustrating pretest and post-test probability of asthma after methacholine challenge test with 4 PC20 values. The curves represent a compilation of information from several sources. They are approximations presented to illustrate the relationships and principles of decision analysis. They are not intended to calculate precise post-test probabilities in patients. (*From* Crapo RO, Casaburi R, Coates AL, et al. Guidelines for methacholine and exercise challenge testing - 1999. Am J Respir Crit Care Med 2000;161(1):309–29; with permission. Copyright © 2000, American Thoracic Society.)

likelihood of having asthma. When a patient presents with symptoms, the pretest probability is expectedly higher, so that if the estimate is between 30% and 70%, a PC20 of 1 mg/mL could bring the post-test estimate to approximately 90% to 98%.

The reported sensitivity and specificity of the methacholine challenge test (MCT) has varied depending on the study population tested. In studies with large sample sizes, sensitivity ranged from 51%[82] to 100%,[83] and specificity ranged from 49%[84] to 100% (**Table 1**).[82–92] Much of these data are based on older clinical trials. However, the current American Thoracic Society (ATS) guidelines suggest that MCTs can be used to exclude asthma if the PC20 is greater than 16 mg/mL in the proper clinical setting.[4] This conclusion was based mainly on studies before inhaled corticosteroids use had become a mainstay treatment for asthma. Hence a negative MCT result has been generally interpreted as indicating that it is unlikely that a patient with respiratory symptoms has asthma. A recent study conducted by the Asthma Clinical Research Consortium demonstrated that in 125 asthmatic subjects receiving controller treatment and 92 nonasthmatic control subjects an MCT, sensitivity of 77% and specificity of 96% were observed with a threshold of 8 mg/mL. Increasing the threshold to 16 mg/mL did not substantially increase the sensitivity.[92] In the latter trial, it was also observed that race and the presence of atopy had a significant effect on methacholine sensitivity. The MCT was much less sensitive in white participants (69%) compared with African Americas (91%, $P = .015$).

There are several issues in cross-comparing the numerous studies evaluating the performance of the MCT. The study population may differ in several ways, racially, in the severity of asthma, in the degree of airflow limitation, the presence or absence of asthma symptoms, presence of underling atopy, and use of controller medications. Finally, it is possible that the method by which the MCT is performed may influence the results. Some previous studies and the ATS guidelines on MCTs have indicated that the 2 MCT methods, 5-breath dosimeter and 2-minute tidal breathing, are equivalent.[93–95] However, 2 groups recently reported evidence of a lack of comparability between the 2 methods.[93,96,97] These authors found that patients with mild asthma (PC20 >2 mg/mL) were more likely to have a positive MCT result with the tidal breathing method than with the 5-breath dosimeter method. Therefore, these variables may explain the disparate results observed in various clinical trials.

Recently, the US Food and Drug Administration approved the dry powder mannitol test for determining BHR in patients 6 years of age or older. Mannitol dry powder is delivered in progressively increasing doses (0, 5, 10, 20, 40, 80, 160, 160, 160 mg), with forced expiratory volume in the first second of expiration (FEV_1) measured 1 minute after each dose. A positive response is a 15% reduction in FEV_1 at a total cumulative dose of 635 mg or a 10% reduction in FEV_1 from baseline between doses. The mannitol test has been suggested for confirming a diagnosis of asthma and to follow response to therapy.[98–102] The advantage of the indirect tests over the direct such as methacholine is that they provide information on 2 key features of asthma, those being airway inflammation and BHR. In addition to a hyper-responsive smooth muscle, a positive response to mannitol or other indirect stimuli indicates both the presence of inflammatory cells, and a sufficient concentration of mediators to cause bronchoconstriction. A negative test result indicates a missing element such as insufficient numbers of inflammatory cells or insufficient concentration of mediators or an unresponsive smooth muscle. Examples of negative tests include known asthmatic patients being treated effectively with inhaled corticosteroids,[103,104] people with eosinophilic bronchitis but no asthma,[105] or people with asymptomatic BHR to methacholine who may have airway injury such as elite athletes.[86,106,107]

Sverrid and colleagues evaluated methacholine and mannitol and reported a specificity of 80.2% (95% CI, 77.1%–82.9%) and 98.4% (95% CI, 96.2%–99.4%),

Table 1
Selected studies evaluating the performance of MCTs

Author (Reference)	Year	Study Population	No.	Adults or Pediatrics	Sensitivity	Specificity	PPV	NPV	Definition of Positive PC$_{20}$ (mg/mL)
Hopp et al[85]	1984	Asthma, healthy control	165	Pediatrics	98%	63%	57%	99%	800 BU[a]
Cockcroft et al[83]	1992	College students	500	Adults	100%	93%	34%	100%	8
Nieminen[88]	1992	Outpatient pulmonary clinic referrals	791	Adults	89%	76%	71%	91%	2600 µg[a]
Perpina et al[89]	1993	Asthma, rhinitis, chronic bronchitis, healthy control	300	Adults	84%	86%	No information	No information	15
Goldstein et al[87]	1994	Allergy clinic referrals	198	Adults, Pediatrics	61%	100%	100%	74%	8
Goldstein et al[91]	2001	Suspected asthmatic patients with normal lung function in private clinic	121	Adults, Pediatrics	86%	100%	100%	56%	8
Liem et al[86]	2008	Manitoba birth cohort: asthma healthy control	640	Pediatrics	66%	64%	No information	No information	4
Anderson et al[82]	2009	Suspected asthmatic patients recruited from multiple study sites	375	Adults, Pediatrics	51%	75%	78%	46%	16
Sverrild et al[90]	2010	Young adults randomly drawn from nation wide registration in Denmark	238	Adults, Pediatrics (age 15-24 y)	69%	80%	49%	90%	8 µ mol[a]
Carlsten et al[84]	2011	Birth cohort with high risk for asthma	348	Pediatrics	80%	49%	27%	92%	3

Abbreviations: BU, Breath units; NPV, negative predictive value; PPV, positive predictive value.
[a] These studies used a provocative dose of methacholine to a positive test results (PD$_{20}$).
(*From* Sumino K, Sugar EA, Irvin CG, et al; American Lung Association Asthma Clinical Research Centers. Methacholine challenge test: Diagnostic characteristics in asthmatic patients receiving controller medications. J Allergy Clin Immunol 2012;130:69-75; with permission).

respectively, with a positive predictive value of 48.6% versus 90.4%, whereas the sensitivity was 68.6% (95% CI, 57.1%–78.4%) and 58.8% (95% CI, 50.7%–62.6%), respectively.[90] Other trials have reported a sensitivity range between 50% and 60%, with specificities in the high 90% range. Although, the sensitivity does not appear to be very high, it is important to recognize that the benefit of current treatment on BHR, a previous diagnosis, or the period of current asthma has not always been taken into account when reporting the data. For example, the sensitivity of mannitol to identify a physician diagnosis of asthma increased from 59.8% to 89% when those taking inhaled steroids and negative to mannitol were excluded.[108]

Overall, the feeling is that mannitol is more sensitive for exercise-induced broncho-spasm than an exercise challenge in detecting BHR, but is not as sensitive as desired for diagnosing exercise induced bronchospasm. However, due to its relatively high specificity, mannitol may serve as a confirmatory test in those with a positive MCT. A comprehensive discussion on this topic is beyond the scope of this article but 2 extensive reviews have been published discussing mannitol challenges.[108,109]

Among asthmatics, in general, an investigation into the relationship between BHR to histamine and exercise illustrated that inhaled direct challenge would be more sensitive than exercise tests at demonstrating increased nonspecific airway reactivity.[110] In that study, 84% of asthmatics had a positive histamine challenge, whereas only half had evidence of a positive exercise test (ie, 10% drop in FEV_1). Despite the high estimate of asthma diagnosis using direct BPCs such as histamine or methacholine in symptomatic patients, this may compare poorly when indirect challenges are used for a specific purpose. For example, a study was undertaken to investigate the relationship between asthma symptoms and BHR to methacholine and eucapnic voluntary hyperpnea (EVH), among symptomatic elite summer-sport athletes because of a notable increase in the prevalence of asthma reports among athletes participating in the Olympic games.[111]

In that study, athletes who reported asthma symptoms were twice as likely to have a positive response to EVH challenge (50%; mean reduction in FEV_1– of 25.4% ± 15%), compared to a positive methacholine challenge (18%; mean PD20 of 1.69 mmol to 2.05 mmol). Although all subjects with positive methacholine challenge results had positive EVH challenge results, methacholine had a negative predictive value of only 61% and a sensitivity of 36% for identifying those responsive to EVH. These results suggest that EVH is a more sensitive test for the diagnosis of BHR in elite athletes, and the differences in response to the direct and indirect stimuli raise the possibility of a different pathogenesis involved.[111]

Airway cooling associated with vigorous physical exercise has been thought of as a presumptive cause of exercise-induced asthma. The association of airway cooling with airway hyper-reactivity is today folded into 2 potential theories: thermal and osmotic hypotheses. Thermal hypothesis refers to cooling of the airways after exercise that is followed by rapid airway warming, which causes vascular congestion, increased permeability, and edema. The osmotic hypothesis implicates evaporated water loss causing hyperosmolality, stimulation of mucosal drying leading to mast cell degranulation, release of inflammatory mediators such as histamine, prostaglandin D2 (PGD2) and the cysteinyl leukotrienes, and ultimately to edema and airway smooth muscle contraction.

Between indirect challenges specifically to hypertonic saline and exercise challenge, the responses to either stimulus seem to track better. From a community-based, cross-sectional survey,[84] 382 children successfully completed a 4.5% hypertonic saline challenge with increasing inhalation periods, and 365 performed a 6-minute standardized, free running exercise challenge. The prevalence of BHR to hypertonic saline was 20.4%. The results showed similar low sensitivity and high specificity values to identify children who had current wheeze, using 4.5% hypertonic saline challenge (47% and 92%, respectively) and a standardized exercise challenge (46% and 88%, respectively). There was a moderate agreement of response to hypertonic saline and to exercise (kappa = 0.43).[112]

There also appear to be differences between direct and indirect stimuli in the evaluation of response to intervention. Patients sensitized to house dust mites who were transferred to a more favorable environment at high altitude demonstrated no significant difference in BHR to methacholine challenge, but developed a significant improvement in airway response to adenosine monophosphate, indicated by displacement of the dose–response curve to the right by 2 doubling concentrations (P = .005) and exercise (P = .03).[77] These results demonstrate the discordance in responses to direct and indirect challenges. The improvement in BHR to the indirect stimuli using adenosine 5'-monophosphate (AMP) and exercise in contrast to the lack of response in BHR to methacholine methacholine suggests amelioration of airway inflammation following avoidance of house dust aeroallergens.[77]

Indirect challenges compared with direct stimuli may also be more sensitive in detecting changes in airway reactivity with inhaled corticosteroid treatment.[67,68,113–116] BHR to methacholine and AMP was compared, as well as induced sputum analysis and exhaled nitric oxide measurements, before and after 2 weeks of treatment with oral or inhaled corticosteroids. Using multiple regression analysis, corticosteroid improvement in AMP PC20 correlated negatively with changes in sputum eosinophils, bronchial epithelial cells, and exhaled nitric oxide, and positively with changes in sputum lymphocytes. On the other hand, improvement in methacholine PC20 correlated negatively with changes in the number of sputum eosniphils and positively with increase in sputum lymphocytes and FEV_1% predicted. There was a stronger correlation between changes in sputum eosinophils and AMP PC20 compared with methacholine PC20 ($r = -0.43$, $P = .0001$ vs $r = -0.28$, $P = .004$, respectively). The total explained variance of the improvement in BHR was greater for changes in AMP compared with changes for methacholine (36% vs 22%, respectively). These suggest that improvement in BHR to adenosine may better detect changes in airway inflammation than improvement in methacholine PC20. After inhalation of an aqueous solution administered as AMP, it is converted immediately to adenosine by the ubiquitous enzyme 5'-nucleotidase. Adenosine exerts its effects on human cells through interaction with specific adenosine (P1) receptors. The exact effects of AMP on airway wall are not well-defined, but the role of mast cells is crucial based on a variety of inflammatory mediators such as histamine, prostaglandins, leukotrienes, and IL-8 release from human mast cells enhanced by adenosine in vitro.[117–120] Although there are studies that have shown differential BHR response to anti-inflammatories such as inhaled corticosteroids, there are also those that show concordant effects of these medications on bronchial responsiveness to direct and indirect stimuli.[104,121–124] Although most of the indirect stimuli that invoke an inflammatory response share a common pathway in the kinetics, the extent to which the initial insult affects the influx of inflammatory cells and release of mediators is what the differential responses between challenges. Perhaps the variability in bronchial response to direct and indirect stimuli from inhaled corticosteroid therapy depends not only on the specific drug or stimulant, but also on the duration of treatment, dosage, and delivery (see **Table 1**).

SUMMARY

BHR is an important feature of asthma, and it is considered a useful tool in the diagnosis, monitoring, and prognostication of a complex condition. With its many valuable uses, it probably represents several inherent elements of the disease process, such as genetic predisposition, airway inflammation, and airway remodeling. Airway inflammation seems to account for the transient and variable component of BHR. Studies of correlations between BHR to direct and indirect stimuli and inflammatory markers, and treatment effects on reduction in BHR and airway inflammation have shown modest associations. The exact mechanisms that explain the association between BHR and airway inflammation are unknown. The permanent or persistent component of BHR, particularly to direct stimuli, correlates significantly with structural changes in the airway, such as basement membrane thickness and epithelial damage. It might be this component that is resistant or refractory to the effects of available interventions. A few trials of specific immunomodulatory therapy have shown considerable improvements in markers of airway inflammation, without significantly modifying airway reactivity. On the other hand, the inflammatory component may explain the variable component that modulates over time and with anti-inflammatory therapy and thus is better reflected by the BHR measured with indirect challenges such as mannitol and exercise. There is certainly a need to develop interventions that will impact the more permanent feature of BHR.

ACKNOWLEDGMENTS

The authors would like to thank Deidre Versluis for her assistance in the preparation of this manuscript.

REFERENCES

1. Joos GF, O'Connor B, Anderson SD, et al. ERS task force indirect airway challenges. Eur Respir J 2003;21(6):1050–68.
2. Peat JK, Toelle BG, Marks GB, et al. Continuing the debate about measuring asthma in population studies. Thorax 2001;56:406–11.
3. Woolcock AJ, Peat JK, Salome CM, et al. Prevalence of bronchial hyperresponsiveness and asthma in a rural adult population. Thorax 1987;42(5):361–8.
4. Crapo RO, Casaburi R, Coates AL, et al. Guidelines for methacholine and exercise challenge testing-1999. This official statement of the American Thoracic Society was adopted by the ATS Board of Directors, July 1999. Am J Respir Crit Care Med 2000;161(1):309–29.
5. Rijcken B, Schouten JP, Weiss ST, et al. Long term variability of bronchial responsiveness to histamine in a random population sample of adults. Am Rev Respir Dis 1993;148:944–94.
6. Cockcroft DW, Berscheid BA, Murdock KY. Unimodal distribution of bronchial responsiveness to inhaled histamine in a random human population. Chest 1983;83(5):751–4.
7. Busse WW, Wanner A, Adams K, et al. Investigative bronchoprovocation and bronchoscopy in airway diseases. Am J Respir Crit Care Med 2005;172(7):807–16.
8. Sont JK, Willems LN, Bel EH, et al. Clinical control and histopathologic outcome of asthma when using airway hyperresponsiveness as an additional guide to long-term treatment. Am J Respir Crit Care Med 1999;159(4 Pt 1):1043–51.
9. Josephs LK, Gregg I, Mullee MA, et al. Nonspecific bronchial reactivity and its relationship to the clinical expression of asthma. A longitudinal study. Am Rev Respir Dis 1989;140:350–7.
10. Weiss ST, Van Natta ML, Zeiger RS. Relationship between increased airway responsiveness and asthma severity in the childhood asthma management program. Am J Respir Crit Care Med 2000;162:50–6.

11. Jansen DF, Schouten JP, Vonk JM, et al. Smoking and airway hyperresponsiveness especially in the presence of blood eosinophilia increase the risk to develop respiratory symptoms: a 25-year follow-up study in the general adult population. Am J Respir Crit Care Med 1999;160:259–64.

12. Carey VJ, Weiss ST, Tager IB, et al. Airways responsiveness, wheeze onset, and recurrent asthma episodes in young adolescents. The East Boston Childhood Respiratory Disease Cohort. Am J Respir Crit Care Med 1996; 153(1):356–61.

13. Rasmussen F, Taylor DR, Flannery EM, et al. Risk factors for airway remodeling in asthma manifested by a low postbronchodilator FEV1/vital capacity ratio: a longitudinal population study from childhood to adulthood. Am J Respir Crit Care Med 2002;165(11):1480–8.

14. Hopp RJ, Bewtra AK, Biven R, et al. Bronchial reactivity pattern in nonasthmatic parents of asthmatics. Ann Allergy 1988;61(3):184–6.

15. Clarke JR, Jenkins MA, Hopper JL, et al. Evidence for genetic associations between asthma, atopy, and bronchial hyperresponsiveness: a study of 8- to 18-yr-old twins. Am J Respir Crit Care Med 2000;162(6):2188–93.

16. Postma DS, Bleecker ER, Amelung PJ, et al. Genetic susceptibility to asthmad-bronchial hyperresponsiveness coinherited with a major gene for atopy. N Engl J Med 1995;333(14):894–900.

17. Ruffilli A, Bonini S. Susceptibility genes for allergy and asthma. Allergy 1997; 52(3):256–73.

18. Marsh DG, Neely JD, Breazeale DR, et al. Linkage analysis of IL4 and other chromosome 5q31.1 markers and total serum immunoglobulin E concentration. Science 1994;264(5162):1152–6.

19. Meyers DA, Postma DS, Stine OC, et al. Genome screen for asthma and bronchial hyper-responsiveness: interactions with passive smoke exposure. J Allergy Clin Immunol 2005;115(6):1169–75.

20. Colilla S, Nicolae D, Pluzhnikov A, et al. Collaborative Study for the Genetics of Asthma. Evidence for gene–environment interactions in a linkage study of asthma and smoking exposure. J Allergy Clin Immunol 2003;111(4):840–6.

21. O'byrne PM, Inman MD. Airway hyperresponsiveness. Chest 2003;123: 411S–6S.

22. Cartier A, Thomson NC, Frith PA, et al. Allergen-induced increase in bronchial responsiveness to histamine: relationship to the late asthmatic response and change in airway caliber. J Allergy Clin Immunol 1982;70(3):170–7.

23. De Monchy JG, Kau.man HF, Venge P, et al. Bronchoalveolar eosinophilia during allergen-induced late asthmatic reactions. Am Rev Respir Dis 1985;131(3): 373–6.

24. Pin I, Freitag AP, O'Byrne PM, et al. Changes in the cellular profile of induced sputum after allergen-induced asthmatic responses. Am Rev Respir Dis 1992; 145(6):1265–9.

25. Metzger WJ, Richerson HB, Worden K, et al. Bronchoalveolar lavage of allergic asthmatic patients following allergen bronchoprovocation. Chest 1986;89(4): 477–83.

26. O'Byrne PM, Walters EH, Gold BD, et al. Neutrophil depletion inhibits airway hyperresponsiveness induced by ozone exposure. Am Rev Respir Dis 1984; 130(2):214–9.

27. Empey DW, Laitinen LA, Jacobs L, et al. Mechanisms of bronchial hyperreactivity in normal subjects after upper respiratory tract infection. Am Rev Respir Dis 1976;113(2):131–9.

28. Laitinen LA, Elkin RB, Empey DW, et al. Bronchial hyperresponsiveness in normal subjects during attenuated influenza virus infection. Am Rev Respir Dis 1991;143(2):358–61.

29. Mapp C, Boschetto P, dal Vecchio L, et al. Protective effect of antiasthma drugs on late asthmatic reactions and increased airway responsiveness induced by toluene diisocyanate in sensitized subjects. Am Rev Respir Dis 1987;136(6):1403–7.

30. Fabbri LM, Boschetto P, Zocca E, et al. Bronchoalveolar neutrophilia during late asthmatic reactions induced by toluene diisocyanate. Am Rev Respir Dis 1987; 136(1):36–42.

31. Jeffery PK, Wardlaw AJ, Nelson FC, et al. Bronchial biopsies in asthma. An ultrastructural, quantitative study and correlation with hyperreactivity. Am Rev Respir Dis 1989;140(6):1745–53.

32. Boulet LP, Laviolette M, Turcotte H, et al. Bronchial subepithelial fibrosis correlates with airway responsiveness to methacholine. Chest 1997;112(1):45–52.

33. Ward C, Pais M, Bish R, et al. Airway inflammation, basement membrane thickening and bronchial hyperresponsiveness in asthma. Thorax 2002;57(4):309–16.

34. Elwood W, Barnes PJ, Chung KF. Airway hyperresponsiveness is associated with inflammatory cell infiltration in allergic brown Norway rats. Int Arch Allergy Immunol 1992;99(1):91–7.

35. Elwood W, Lötvall JO, Barnes PJ, et al. Characterization of allergen-induced bronchial hyperresponsiveness and airway inflammation in actively sensitized brown-Norway rats. J Allergy Clin Immunol 1991;88(6):951–60.

36. Boulet LP, Cartier A, Thomson NC, et al. Asthma and increases in nonallergic bronchial responsiveness from seasonal pollen exposure. J Allergy Clin Immunol 1983;71(4):399–406.

37. Palmqvist M, Pettersson K, Sjöstrand M, et al. Mild experimental exacerbation of asthma induced by individualised low-dose repeated allergen exposure. A double-blind evaluation. Respir Med 1998;92(10):1223–30.

38. Hessel EM, Van Oosterhout AJ, Van Ark I, et al. Development of airway hyperresponsiveness is dependent on interferon-gamma and independent of eosinophil infiltration. Am J Respir Cell Mol Biol 1997;16(3):325–34.

39. Wilder JA, Collie DD, Wilson BS, et al. Dissociation of airway hyperresponsiveness from immunoglobulin E and airway eosinophilia in a murine model of allergic asthma. Am J Respir Cell Mol Biol 1999;20(6):1326–34.

40. De Sanctis GT, Itoh A, Green FH, et al. T-lymphocytes regulate genetically determined airway hyperresponsiveness in mice. Nat Med 1997;3(4):460–2.

41. Gavett SH, Chen X, Finkelman F, et al. Depletion of murine CD4pT lymphocytes prevents antigen-induced airway hyperreactivity and pulmonary eosinophilia. Am J Respir Cell Mol Biol 1994;10(6):587–93.

42. Krinzman SJ, De Sanctis GT, Cernadas M, et al. Inhibition of T cell costimulation abrogates airway hyperresponsiveness in a murine model. J Clin Invest 1996; 98(12):2693–9.

43. Kamachi A, Nasuhara Y, Nishimura M, et al. Dissociation between airway responsiveness to methacholine and responsiveness to antigen. Eur Respir J 2002;19(1):76–83.

44. Ferguson AC, Wong FW. Bronchial hyperresponsiveness in asthmatic children. Correlation with macrophages and eosinophils in broncholavage fluid. Chest 1989;96:988–91.

45. Gibson PG, Saltos N, Borgas T. Airway mast cells and eosinophils correlate with clinical severity and airway hyperresponsiveness in corticosteroid-treated asthma. J Allergy Clin Immunol 2000;105(4):752–9.

46. Kelly C, Ward C, Stenton CS, et al. Number and activity of inflammatory cells in bronchoalveolar lavage fluid in asthma and their relation to airway responsiveness. Thorax 1988;43:684–92.
47. Heaton T, Rowe J, Turner S, et al. An immunoepidemiological approach to asthma: identification of in-vitro T-cell response patterns associated with different wheezing phenotypes in children. Lancet 2005;365(9454):142–9.
48. Kirby JG, Hargreave FE, Gleich GJ, et al. Bronchoalveolar cell profiles of asthmatic and nonasthmatic subjects. Am Rev Respir Dis 1987;136(2):379–83.
49. Wardlaw AJ, Dunnette S, Gleich GJ, et al. Eosinophils and mast cells in bronchoalveolar lavage in subjects with mild asthma. Relationship to bronchial hyperreactivity. Am Rev Respir Dis 1988;137(1):62–9.
50. Pliss LB, Ingenito EP, Ingram RH Jr. Responsiveness, inflammation, and effects of deep breaths on obstruction in mild asthma. J Appl Physiol 1989;66(5):2298–304.
51. Woolley KL, Adelroth E, Woolley MJ, et al. Granulocyte-macrophage colony-stimulating factor, eosinophils and eosinophil cationic protein in subjects with and without mild, stable, atopic asthma. Eur Respir J 1994;7(9):1576–84.
52. Bradley BL, Azzawi M, Jacobson M, et al. Eosinophils, T-lymphocytes, mast cells, neutrophils, and macrophages in bronchial biopsy specimens from atopic subjects with asthma: comparison with biopsy specimens from atopic subjects without asthma and normal control subjects and relationship to bronchial hyper-responsiveness. J Allergy Clin Immunol 1991;88(4):661–74.
53. Chetta A, Foresi A, Del Donno M, et al. Bronchial responsiveness to distilled water and methacholine and its relationship to inflammation and remodeling of the airways in asthma. Am J Respir Crit Care Med 1996;153:910–7.
54. Pin I, Radford S, Kolendowicz R, et al. Airway inflammation in symptomatic and asymptomatic children with methacholine hyperresponsiveness. Eur Respir J 1993;6(9):1249–56.
55. Pizzichini E, Pizzichini MM, Efthimiadis A, et al. Indices of airway inflammation in induced sputum: reproducibility and validity of cell and fluid-phase measurements. Am J Respir Crit Care Med 1996;154(2 Pt 1):308–17.
56. Foresi A, Leone C, Pelucchi A, et al. Eosinophils, mast cells, and basophils in induced sputum from patients with seasonal allergic rhinitis and perennial asthma: relationship to methacholine responsiveness. J Allergy Clin Immunol 1997;100(1):58–64.
57. Jansen DF, Rijcken B, Schouten JP, et al. The relationship of skin test positivity, high serum total IgE levels, and peripheral blood eosinophilia to symptomatic and asymptomatic airway hyperresponsiveness. Am J Respir Crit Care Med 1999;159(3):924–31.
58. Jatakanon A, Lim S, Kharitonov SA, et al. Correlation between exhaled nitric oxide, sputum eosinophils, and methacholine responsiveness in patients with mild asthma. Thorax 1998;53(2):91–5.
59. Reid DW, Johns DP, Feltis B, et al. Exhaled nitric oxide continues to reflect airway hyper-responsiveness and disease activity in inhaled corticosteroid-treated adult asthmatic patients. Respirology 2003;8(4):479–86.
60. Chan-Yeung M, Leriche J, Maclean L, et al. Comparison of cellular and protein changes in bronchial lavage fluid of symptomatic and asymptomatic patients with red cedar asthma on follow-up examination. Clin Allergy 1988;18(4):359–65.
61. Djukanović R, Wilson JW, Britten KM, et al. Quantitation of mast cells and eosinophils in the bronchial mucosa of symptomatic atopic asthmatics and healthy control subjects using immunohistochemistry. Am Rev Respir Dis 1990;142(4):863–71.

62. Adelroth E, Rosenhall L, Johansson SA, et al. Inflammatory cells and eosinophilic activity in asthmatics investigated by bronchoalveolar lavage. The effects of antiasthmatic treatment with budesonide or terbutaline. Am Rev Respir Dis 1990;142(1):91–9.
63. Ollerenshaw SL, Woolcock AJ. Characteristics of the inflammation in biopsies from large airways of subjects with asthma and subjects with chronic airflow limitation. Am Rev Respir Dis 1992;145(4 Pt 1):922–7.
64. Iredale MJ, Wanklyn SA, Phillips IP, et al. Non-invasive assessment of bronchial inflammation in asthma: no correlation between eosinophilia of induced sputum and bronchial responsiveness to inhaled hypertonic saline. Clin Exp Allergy 1994;24(10):940–5.
65. Crimi E, Spanevello A, Neri M, et al. Dissociation between airway inflammation and airway hyperresponsiveness in allergic asthma. Am J Respir Crit Care Med 1998;157(1):4–9.
66. Oddera S, Silvestri M, Penna R, et al. Airway eosinophilic inflammation and bronchial hyperresponsiveness after allergen inhalation challenge in asthma. Lung 1998;176(4):237–47.
67. Meijer RJ, Kerstjens HA, Arends LR, et al. Effects of inhaled fluticasone and oral prednisolone on clinical and inflammatory parameters in patients with asthma. Thorax 1999;54(10):894–9.
68. Nielsen KG, Bisgaard H. The effect of inhaled budesonide on symptoms, lung function, and cold air and methacholine responsiveness in 2-to 5-year-old asthmatic children. Am J Respir Crit Care Med 2000;162(4 Pt 1):1500–6.
69. van den Berge M, Kerstjens HA, Meijer RJ, et al. Corticosteroid-induced improvement in the PC20 of adenosine monophosphate is more closely associated with reduction in airway inflammation than improvement in the PC20 of methacholine. Am J Respir Crit Care Med 2001;164(7):1127–32.
70. The Childhood Asthma Management Program Research Group. Long-term effects of budesonide or nedocromil in children with asthma. N Engl J Med 2000;343(15):1054–63.
71. Juniper EF, Kline PA, Vanzieleghem MA, et al. Effect of long-term treatment with an inhaled corticosteroid (budesonide) on airway hyperresponsiveness and clinical asthma in nonsteroid-dependent asthmatics. Am Rev Respir Dis 1990;142:832–6.
72. Kerrebijn KF, van Essen-Zandvliet EE, Neijens HJ. Effect of long-term treatment with inhaled corticosteroids and beta-agonists on the bronchial responsiveness in children with asthma. J Allergy Clin Immunol 1987;79:653–9.
73. Bisgaard H, Nielsen KG. Bronchoprotection with a leukotriene receptor antagonist in asthmatic preschool children. Am J Respir Crit Care Med 2000;162(1):187–90.
74. Le JA, Busse WW, Pearlman D, et al. Montelukast, a leukotriene-receptor antagonist, for the treatment of mild asthma and exercise-induced bronchoconstriction. N Engl J Med 1998;339(3):147–52.
75. Le JA. Leukotriene modifiers as novel therapeutics in asthma. Clin Exp Allergy 1998;28(Suppl 5):147–53.
76. Fischer AR, McFadden CA, Frantz R, et al. Effect of chronic 5-lipoxygenase inhibition on airway hyperresponsiveness in asthmatic subjects. Am J Respir Crit Care Med 1995;152:1203–7.
77. Benckhuijsen J, van den Bos JW, van Velzen E, et al. Differences in the effect of allergen avoidance on bronchial hyperresponsiveness as measured by methacholine, adenosine 5'monophosphate, and exercise in asthmatic children. Pediatr Pulmonol 1996;22(3):147–53.

78. van Velzen E, van den Bos JW, Benckhuijsen JA, et al. Effect of allergen avoidance at high altitude on direct and indirect bronchial hyperresponsiveness and markers of inflammation in children with allergic asthma. Thorax 1996;51(6):582–4.
79. Leckie MJ, ten Brinke A, Khan J, et al. Effects of an interleukin-5 blocking monoclonal antibody on eosinophils, airway hyperresponsiveness, and the late asthmatic response. Lancet 2000;356(9248):2144–8.
80. Djukanović R, Wilson SJ, Kraft M, et al. Effects of treatment with anti-immunoglobulin E antibody omalizumab on airway inflammation in allergic asthma. Am J Respir Crit Care Med 2004;170(6):583–93.
81. Juniper EF, Frith PA, Dunnett C, et al. Reproducibility and comparison of responses to inhaled histamine and methacholine. Thorax 1978;33:705–10.
82. Anderson SD, Charlton B, Weiler JM, et al. Comparison of mannitol and methacholine to predict exercise-induced bronchoconstriction and a clinical diagnosis of asthma. Respir Res 2009;10:4.
83. Cockcroft DW, Murdock KY, Berscheid BA, et al. Sensitivity and specificity of histamine PC20 determination in a random selection of young college students. J Allergy Clin Immunol 1992;89:23–30.
84. Carlsten C, Dimich-Ward H, Ferguson A, et al. Airway hyperresponsiveness to methacholine in 7-year-old children: sensitivity and specificity for pediatric allergist-diagnosed asthma. Pediatr Pulmonol 2011;46:175–8.
85. Hopp RJ, Bewtra AK, Nair NM, et al. Specificity and sensitivity of methacholine inhalation challenge in normal and asthmatic children. J Allergy Clin Immunol 1984;74:154–8.
86. Liem JJ, Kozyrskyj AL, Cockroft DW, et al. Diagnosing asthma in children: what is the role for methacholine bronchoprovocation testing? Pediatr Pulmonol 2008;43:481–9.
87. Goldstein MF, Pacana SM, Dvorin DJ, et al. Retrospective analyses of methacholine inhalation challenges. Chest 1994;105:1082–8.
88. Nieminen MM. Unimodal distribution of bronchial hyperresponsiveness to methacholine in asthmatic patients. Chest 1992;102:1537–43.
89. Perpina M, Pellicer C, de Diego A, et al. Diagnostic value of the bronchial provocation test with methacholine in asthma. A Bayesian analysis approach. Chest 1993;104:149–54.
90. Sverrild A, Porsbjerg C, Thomsen SF, et al. Airway hyperresponsiveness to mannitol and methacholine and exhaled nitric oxide: a random-sample population study. J Allergy Clin Immunol 2010;126:952–8.
91. Goldstein MF, Veza BA, Dunsky EH, et al. Comparisons of peak diurnal expiratory flow variation, postbronchodilator FEV(1) responses, and methacholine inhalation challenges in the evaluation of suspected asthma. Chest 2001;119:1001–10.
92. Sumino K, Sugar EA, Irvin CG, et al, American Lung Association Asthma Clinical Research Centers. Methacholine challenge test: diagnostic characteristics in asthmatic patients receiving controller medications. J Allergy Clin Immunol 2012;130:69–75.
93. Prieto L, Ferrer A, Domenech J, et al. Effect of challenge method on sensitivity, reactivity, and maximal response to methacholine. Ann Allergy Asthma Immunol 2006;97:175–81.
94. Wubbel C, Asmus MJ, Stevens G, et al. Methacholine challenge testing: comparison of the two American Thoracic Society-recommended methods. Chest 2004;125:453–8.
95. Siersted HC, Walker CM, O'Shaughnessy AD, et al. Comparison of two standardized methods of methacholine inhalation challenge in young adults. Eur Respir J 2000;15:181–4.

96. Cockcroft DW, Davis BE, Todd DC, et al. Methacholine challenge: comparison of two methods. Chest 2005;127(3):839–44.

97. Cockcroft DW. Methacholine challenge methods. Chest 2008;134:678–80.

98. Cockcroft D, Davis B. Direct and indirect challenges in the clinical assessment of asthma. Ann Allergy Asthma Immunol 2009;103:363–70.

99. Cockcroft DW. Direct challenge tests. Chest 2010;138:18S–24S.

100. Porsbjerg C, Brannan JD, Anderson SD, et al. Relationship between airway responsiveness to mannitol and to methacholine and markers of airway inflammation, peak flow variability and quality of life in asthma patients. Clin Exp Allergy 2008;38:43–50.

101. Porsbjerg C, Backer V, Joos G, et al. Current and future use of the mannitol bronchial challenge in everyday clinical practice. Clin Respir J 2009;3:189–97.

102. Brannan JD, Koskela H, Anderson SD. Monitoring asthma therapy using indirect bronchial provocation tests. Clin Respir J 2007;1:3–15.

103. Leuppi JD, Salome CM, Jenkins CR, et al. Predictive markers of asthma exacerbations during stepwise dose reduction of inhaled corticosteroids. Am J Respir Crit Care Med 2001;163:406–12.

104. Koskela HO, Hyvärinen L, Brannan JD, et al. Sensitivity and validity of three bronchial provocation tests to demonstrate the effect of inhaled corticosteroids in asthma. Chest 2003;124:1341–9.

105. Singapuri A, McKenna S, Brightling CE, et al. Mannitol and AMP do not induce bronchoconstriction in eosinophilic bronchitis: further evidence for disassociation between airway inflammation and bronchial hyperresponsiveness. Respirology 2010;15:510–5.

106. Sue-Chu M, Brannan JD, Anderson SD, et al. Airway hyperresponsiveness to methacholine, adenosine5-monophosphate, mannitol, eucapnic voluntary hyperpnoea and field exercise challenge in elite cross country skiers. Br J Sports Med 2010;44:827–32.

107. Porsbjerg C, Rasmussen L, Thomsen SF, et al. Response to mannitol in asymptomatic subjects with airway hyper-responsiveness to methacholine. Clin Exp Allergy 2007;37:22–8.

108. Anderson SD, Brannan JD. Bronchial provocation testing: the future. Curr Opin Allergy Clin Immunol 2011;11(1):46–52.

109. Anderson SD. Indirect challenge tests: airway hyperresponsiveness in asthma: its measurement and clinical significance. Chest 2010;138(Suppl 2):25S–30S.

110. Anderton RC, Cu MT, Frith PA, et al. Bronchial responsiveness to inhaled histamine and exercise. J Allergy Clin Immunol 1979;63:315–20.

111. Holzer K, Anderson SD, Douglass J. Exercise in elite summer athletes: challenges for diagnosis. J Allergy Clin Immunol 2002;110:374–80.

112. Riedler J, Reade T, Dalton M, et al. Hypertonic saline challenge in an epidemiologic survey of asthma in children. Am J Respir Crit Care Med 1994;150: 1632–9.

113. O'Connor BJ, Ridge SM, Barnes PJ, et al. Greater effect of inhaled budesonide on adenosine 5'-monophosphate-induced than on sodium-metabisulfite-induced bronchoconstriction in asthma. Am Rev Respir Dis 1992;146:560–4.

114. Doull IJ, Sandall D, Smith S, et al. Differential inhibitory effect of regular inhaled corticosteroid on airway responsiveness to adenosine 5' monophosphate, methacholine, and bradykinin in symptomatic children with recurrent wheeze. Pediatr Pulmonol 1997;23:404–11.

115. Weersink EJ, Douma RR, Postma DS, et al. Flflucatisone propionate, salmeterol xinafoate, and their combination in the treatment of nocturnal asthma. Am J Respir Crit Care Med 1997;155:1241–6.
116. Reynolds CJ, Togias A, Proud D. Airways hyperresponsiveness to bradykinin and methacholine: effects of inhaled flucatisone. Clin Exp Allergy 2002;32:1174–9.
117. Church MK, Holgate ST, Hughes PJ. Adenosine inhibits and potentiates IgE-dependent histamine release from human basophils by an A2-receptor mediated mechanism. Br J Pharmacol 1983;80:719–26.
118. Hughes PJ, Holgate ST, Church MK. Adenosine inhibits and potentiates IgE-dependent histamine release from human lung mast cells by an A2-purinoceptor mediated mechanism. Biochem Pharmacol 1984;33:3847–52.
119. Peachell PT, Columbo M, Kagey-Sobotka A, et al. Adenosine potentiates mediator release from human lung mast cells. Am Rev Respir Dis 1988;138:1143–51.
120. Forsythe P, McGarvey LP, Heaney LG, et al. Adenosine induces histamine release from human bronchoalveolar lavage mast cells. Clin Sci 1999;96:349–55.
121. Fuller RW, Choudry NB, Eriksson G. Action of budesonide on asthmatic bronchial hyper-responsiveness: effects on directly and indirectly acting bronchoconstrictors. Chest 1991;100:670–4.
122. Vathenen AS, Knox AJ, Wisniewski A, et al. Effect of inhaled budesonide on bronchial reactivity to histamine, exercise, and eucapnic dry air in patients with asthma. Thorax 1991;46:811–6.
123. Rodwell LT, Anderson SD, Seale JP. Inhaled steroids modify bronchial responses to hyper-osmolar saline. Eur Respir J 1992;5:953–62.
124. du Toit JI, Anderson SD, Jenkins CR, et al. Airway responsiveness in asthma: bronchial challenge with histamine and 4.5% sodium chloride before and after budesonide. Allergy Asthma Proc 1997;18:7–14.

Urinary leukotriene E_4 as a Biomarker of Exposure, Susceptibility and Risk in Asthma

Nathan Rabinovitch, MD, MPH

KEYWORDS

- Urinary leukotriene E_4 • Montelukast • Cysteinyl leukotriene • Second hand smoke

KEY POINTS

- Measurement of urinary LTE_4 ($uLTE_4$) can be a useful noninvasive method to assess changes in the rate of total body cysteinyl leukotriene levels.
- The P2Y12 receptor may be important in mediating LTE_4- related airway inflammation.
- $uLTE_4$ is a biomarker of exposure to both atopic and non-atopic asthma triggers such as air pollution and second hand smoke (SHS).
- High $uLTE_4$ levels may be a marker of increased susceptibility to SHS in children with asthma.
- The ratio of $uLTE_4$ to fractional exhaled nitric oxide is associated with a better response to leukotriene receptor antagonist than to inhaled corticosteroid treatment in children with mild to moderate asthma.

LEUKOTRIENE E_4 SYNTHESIS

Urinary leukotriene E_4 ($uLTE_4$) is a biomarker of total body cysteinyl leukotriene (CysLT) production and excretion. Leukotrienes are a family of lipid mediators derived from arachidonic acid through the 5-lipoxygenase pathway. They are produced by various leukocytes, hence the first part of their name (leuko). The triene part of the name refers to the number (3) of conjugated double bonds (alkenes). The first leukotriene to be synthesized, leukotriene A4 (LTA_4), is formed through the conversion of arachidonic acid, located in membrane phospholipids, to 5-hydroperoxyeicosatetraenoic and LTA_4 through membrane-bound 5-lipoxygenase (5-LO) and 5-lipoxygenase–activating protein (FLAP). The 5-LO inhibitor zileuton blocks this conversion step. In human mast cells, basophils, eosinophils, and macrophages, LTA_4 converts quickly either to LTB_4 (through leukotriene hydrolase) or LTC_4 by LTC_4 synthase with the incorporation of glutathione (g-glutamyl-cysteinyl-glycine). LTC_4 is subsequently converted to LTD_4 and then to the stable end product LTE_4. Because of the incorporation of cysteine, LTC_4, LTD_4, and LTE_4 are called cysteinyl leukotrienes (CysLTs) (**Fig. 1**).[1]

This article was supported by NIH ES015510-01.

Department of Pediatrics, National Jewish Health, 1400 Jackson Street, Denver, CO 80206, USA

E-mail address: rabinovitchn@njhealth.org

Immunol Allergy Clin N Am 32 (2012) 433–445

http://dx.doi.org/10.1016/j.iac.2012.06.012

0889-8561/12/$ – see front matter © 2012 Elsevier Inc. All rights reserved.

immunology.theclinics.com

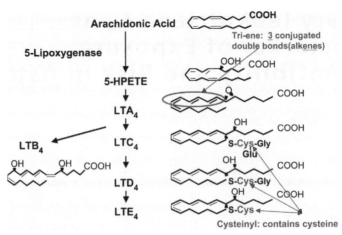

Fig. 1. The major steps in CysLT formation. 5-HPETE, 5-hydroperoxyeicosatetraenoic acid.

CYSTEINYL LEUKOTRIENE RECEPTORS

Both the cysteinyl leukotriene 1 receptor (CysLTR1) and CysLTR2 are constitutively expressed and unregulated in milieus with high cytokine levels.[2–6] CysLTR1 is expressed primarily on blood leukocytes such as monocytes/macrophages, eosinophils, basophils, mast cells, neutrophils, T and B lymphocytes, and on interstitial cells of the nasal mucosa and airway smooth muscle (**Fig. 2**).[3–5] The cellular distribution of CysLTR1 suggests a positive feedback loop because many cells that express CysLT1R also synthesize CysLTs. Leukotriene receptor antagonists (LTRA) such as montelukast block CysLTR1 but not CysLTR2. CysLTR2 is highly expressed in heart

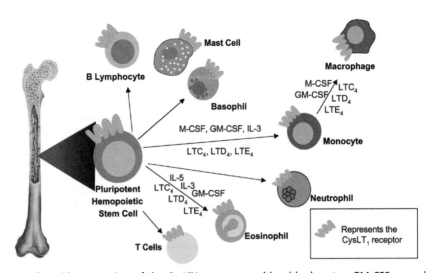

Fig. 2. The wide expression of the CysLT1 receptor on blood leukocytes. GM-CSF, granulocyte-macrophage colony-stimulating factor; M-CSF, macrophage-specific colony-stimulating factor. (*Adapted from* Figueroa DJ, Breyer RM, Defoe SK, et al. Expression of the cysteinyl leukotriene 1 receptor in normal human lung and peripheral blood leukocytes. Am J Respir Crit Care Med 2001;163:232, and Merck Inc; with permission.)

tissue, coronary vessels, and different regions of the brain, with lower expression in peripheral blood cells.[7-9] Although unique functional characteristics of each receptor have not yet been clearly defined,[6] the differential distribution may indicate a greater role for CysLTs acting through CysLTR2 in cardiovascular diseases. Of the 3 CysLT isoforms (LTC$_4$, LTD$_4$, and LTE$_4$), LTE$_4$ has the weakest affinity for CysLTR1 and CysLTR2. As such, LTE$_4$ was thought of as a marker of CysLT formation and effect but not necessarily an important biologic mediator in disease pathogenesis. In a report published in 2009, Paruchuri and colleagues[10] reported that LTE$_4$ potentiated the severity of ovalbumin-induced eosinophilic inflammation in sensitized mice lacking CysLTR1 and CysLTR2, suggesting that there was an additional receptor that could interact with LTE$_4$. These researchers identified the purigenic receptor P2Y12, which binds adenosine diphosphate (ADP) and is expressed primarily on platelets as being necessary for these LTE$_4$-mediated effects, although direct binding between LTE$_4$ and the P2Y12 receptor was not observed. Although the mechanisms of interaction and clinical implications of this novel finding are presently unclear, the potential for cross talk between the purigenic and CysLT pathways is intriguing.

MEASUREMENT OF uLTE$_4$

Measurement of uLTE$_4$ can be a useful noninvasive method to assess changes in the rate of total body CysLT levels. Levels of LTE$_4$ are too low to measure in serum[11,12] but can be measured after excretion into the urine. Studies have shown that inhalation of LTC$_4$ or LTD$_4$ leads to a dose-dependant increase in uLTE$_4$.[13] Approximately 5% of airway CysLTs are eventually eliminated in the urine,[14] almost all in the form of uLTE$_4$, with little if any measurable urinary LTC$_4$ or LTD$_4$.[15]

Various methods for detection of uLTE$_4$ have been reported, including mass spectrometry and radioimmunoassay. Enzyme immunoassays have been shown to be a sensitive method for measuring uLTE$_4$.[16] Although correlations are good, absolute levels tend to be biased high compared with measurements after solid-phase extraction and reverse-phase high-performance liquid chromatography, indicating poor antibody specificity.[17,18] Therefore, enzyme immunoassays may overestimate uLTE$_4$ measurements. Enrichment procedures to further purify the urine have been devised that increase the specificity of the immunoassay,[18] although these techniques are labor intensive and costly. New high-throughput and less labor-intensive methods for measuring uLTE$_4$ based on automated sample enrichment and liquid chromatography/tandem mass spectrometry have now been developed that have lower coefficients of variation and almost 100% recovery using spiked samples, indicating high sensitivity and precision.[19,20] Measurements are often reported in picogram (pg) amounts per milligram (mg) of creatinine to control for urine dilution.

SOURCES OF uLTE$_4$ VARIABILITY

Because no standardized methodology currently exists, reported values for basal uLTE$_4$ levels in healthy individuals vary depending on the measurement technique and whether purification techniques are used in immunoassays. Based on several studies using different assay methodology, uLTE$_4$ levels seem to be partly age related. Mean uLTE$_4$ levels measured by immunoassay with purification in healthy children aged 3 to 12 years were higher than those for healthy adults, measuring 103 pg/mg compared with 80 pg/mg, respectively.[18] Using a mass spectrometry assay with on-line purification uLTE$_4$ values in healthy adults ranged from 17.2 to 63.0 pg/mg and averaged 36.7 pg/mg, whereas uLTE$_4$ values for healthy children ranged from 9.0 to 115.1 pg/mg and averaged 50.7 pg/mg.[19] In contrast, uLTE$_4$ levels may increase with age in adults who have asthma.[21] Genetic polymorphisms within the leukotriene synthesis pathway may also be a source of individual variation,[22] although the modifying effect of these polymorphisms may be seen only after challenges that result in increased uLTE$_4$ levels. Bizzintino and colleagues[23] compared uLTE$_4$ levels during and after asthma exacerbation and reported that increases were related to expression of single-nucleotide polymorphisms (SNP) in the LTC$_4$ synthase (LTC$_4$S-444A) and cysteinyl leukotriene receptor 1 gene (CYSLTR1-927T). Di Lorenzo and colleagues[24] reported that increases in uLTE$_4$ levels after aspirin challenge varied by expression of the cyclooxygenase-1 22 SNP. Because a variety of exposures may increase uLTE$_4$ levels (discussed later), gene interactions may differ depending on the type of environmental challenge and the pathway being studied.

uLTE$_4$ AS A MARKER OF CYsLT-MEDIATED DISEASES

Because many inflammatory mediators, including multiple cytokines, induce CysLT production, high uLTE$_4$ levels may indicate a heightened inflammatory state but do not necessarily suggest that CysLTs are important mediators of a particular disease or that treatment with leukotriene modifiers would be effective. Increased levels of uLTE$_4$ have been reported after episodes of unstable angina and acute myocardial infarction,[25] in coronary artery disease,[26] after coronary artery bypass surgery,[27] and in patients who have atopic dermatitis,[28] rheumatoid arthritis,[29] Crohn disease,[30] and malignant astrocytoma.[31] There are no randomized studies showing that leukotriene-modifying medications are effective treatments for any of these diseases.

The significance of CysLTs as key mediators and modulators in the pathogenesis of asthma is better defined than for other diseases. Inhaled LTD$_4$ is a bronchoconstrictor that is 10,000 times more potent than histamine or methacholine.[32,33] In addition to their potent bronchoconstrictive properties, CysLTs induce other pathophysiologic responses characteristic of the inflammatory response in asthma. As the first step in the allergic response, antibody-presenting dendritic cells track from peripheral tissues to lymph nodes; this movement is enhanced in the presence of CysLTs.[34] LTD$_4$ acts synergistically with other cytokines to increase the proliferation of eosinophils in the bone marrow and peripheral blood[35] and to facilitate eosinophil recruitment into the airway by acting as a chemoattractant and increasing levels of adhesion molecules such as P-selectin.[36,37] In addition, CysLTs reduce eosinophil apoptosis and increase the production of mediators, such as interleukin 5, that increase eosinophil survival (**Fig. 3**).[38,39] Vasodilation and increased microvascular permeability leading to tissue edema and increased airway responsiveness to histamine are also associated with increases in CysLTs.[40,41] CysLTs may also play a role in structural changes in the airway that accompany chronic asthma, such as airway smooth muscle proliferation and remodeling.[42,43] In this context, an assessment of the relationship between exposure to specific asthma triggers and increases in uLTE$_4$ levels can help elucidate the relative importance of CysLTs as mediators of asthma exacerbation. Increased uLTE$_4$ levels are seen with early allergen-induced bronchoconstriction[44] and within 4 hours of exercise, returning to baseline within 24 hours.[45] These postchallenge health effects are at least partially blocked by LTRAs.[45] uLTE$_4$ levels are also increased with exposure to particulate air pollution[46] (**Fig. 4**), tobacco smoke exposure,[47] and upper respiratory infections. Piedimonte and colleagues[48] reported that uLTE$_4$ was 8-fold higher in infants who had bronchiolitis than in controls, and was particularly increased in young infants who had an atopic/asthmatic background. Takahashi and colleagues[49] observed increased uLTE$_4$ levels in children infected with respiratory syncytial virus independently of atopic status. These associations support a clinical study that

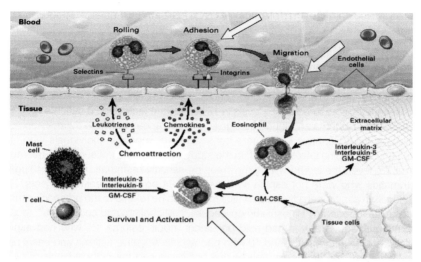

Fig. 3. The multiple in vitro effects of CysLTs on eosinophils. (*From* Rothenberg ME. Eosinophilia. N Engl J Med 1998;338:1594; with permission.)

reported decreased viral-induced asthma exacerbations in children treated with LTRAs.[50]

EFFECT OF ASTHMA CONTROLLER MEDICATIONS ON uLTE$_4$ LEVELS

Studies suggest at least some inhibition of cysteinyl leukotriene formation and uLTE$_4$ excretion with inhaled corticosteroid (ICS) use.[51,52] However, this inhibition does not seem to weaken the ability of uLTE$_4$ to discriminate between patients with and without asthma-related airway inflammation.[53] This relative steroid insensitivity may be an attractive feature of uLTE$_4$ compared with other biomarkers, such as fractional exhaled nitric oxide (FE$_{NO}$), that are exquisitely sensitive to changes in oral or inhaled corticosteroid use.[54] In a study of adults who had mild to moderate asthma, the 5-LO inhibitor zileuton increased asthma control and decreased uLTE$_4$ levels by approximately 40%,[55] suggesting that a modest decrease in leukotriene production may still result in clinically significant improvements in asthma severity. In contrast, use of LTRAs in patients who had asthma did not significantly change uLTE$_4$ levels in 2 placebo-controlled studies.[56,57]

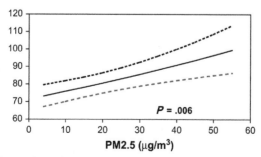

Fig. 4. uLTE$_4$ as a biomarker of ambient particulate air pollution. Regression and standard error lines for the relationship between uLTE$_4$ levels and ambient concentrations of particles less than 2.5 μm (PM2.5) in diameter measured on the same day.

uLTE$_4$ AS A MARKER OF ASTHMA PREVALENCE AND SEVERITY

Some, but not all, studies have reported higher uLTE$_4$ levels in patients with asthma. Asano and colleagues[58] measured 16 consecutive 4-hour urine samples in 5 normal subjects and 8 who had asthma. Mean uLTE$_4$ levels were 84 pg/mg in healthy subjects and 110 pg/mg in asthmatics. Similar differences between individuals with and without asthma were reported by Yamamoto and colleagues[59] and Suzuki and colleagues.[60] In contrast, Smith and colleagues[61] measured uLTE$_4$ levels in 17 healthy subjects and 28 patients with non–aspirin-sensitive asthma and found no significant differences between them.

Increases in uLTE$_4$ have been more consistently observed in individuals who have asthma and are aspirin intolerant.[61–63] In the study by Smith and colleagues,[61] geometric mean uLTE$_4$ levels measured 101 pg/mg in aspirin-sensitive asthmatic patients, 43 pg/mg in asthmatics who were not aspirin sensitive, and 34 pg/mg in healthy subjects. High uLTE$_4$ levels in aspirin-sensitive asthmatics might also be related to the presence of nasal polyposis, as reported by Higashi and colleagues.[64] Micheletto and colleagues[65] studied 34 normal subjects, 39 who had mild persistent atopic asthma, 24 who had aspirin-sensitive asthma with rhinitis, and 10 who had aspirin-sensitive asthma and nasal polyposis. Subjects who had asthma and nasal polyposis had the highest levels of uLTE$_4$ (432 pg/mg) compared with those who had asthma with rhinitis (330 pg/mg), those who had mild persistent asthma (129 pg/mg), and healthy controls (66 pg/mg).

Baseline uLTE$_4$ levels have been associated not only with the presence of asthma but also with disease severity in some, but not all, studies. Vachier and colleagues[66] measured uLTE$_4$ in 40 patients who had severe asthma, 25 patients who had mild to moderate asthma, and 20 nonasthmatic controls. uLTE$_4$ levels were higher in patients with severe asthma (69 pg/mg) compared with patients with mild to moderate asthma (45 pg/mg) and with healthy controls (42 pg/mg). In contrast, a study of 168 patients by Misso and colleagues[21] observed significantly reduced uLTE$_4$ levels in patients who had severe asthma compared with mild or moderate asthmatics.

Studies have also reported associations between uLTE$_4$ and indices of asthma severity, such as lung function parameters, biomarkers of inflammation, or symptoms. Severien and colleagues[52] reported significant differences in uLTE$_4$ levels in children with mild to severe asthma (median 238 pg/mg) compared with healthy nonasthmatic children (189 pg/mg). Associations were also seen between levels of uLTE$_4$ and intra-thoracic gas volume, residual volume, forced expiratory volume in 1 second (FEV$_1$), and forced expiratory capacity (FVC).

Several studies have suggested that within-subject variability in uLTE$_4$ levels is associated with decreased asthma control. Kurokawa and colleagues[67] measured uLTE$_4$ every 3 hours in patients who had asthma with and without nocturnal symptoms and reported that levels from 3:00 AM to 6:00 AM were significantly higher than from 3:00 PM to 6:00 PM in individuals who had nocturnal symptoms, but not in non-nocturnal asthmatics. These investigators suggested that nocturnal asthma symptoms might be related to nighttime spikes in CysLT production, although uLTE$_4$ could also have been a marker for other mediators that co-vary with CysLTs. Similar findings were reported by Bellia and colleagues.[68] These small studies with repeated measurements support the usefulness of measuring within-subject changes in uLTE$_4$ as sensitive predictors of asthma control. In a similar context, Rabinovitch and colleagues[69] followed 50 schoolchildren with primarily moderate to severe asthma over 5 months and reported that within-subject uLTE$_4$ changes were associated with FEV$_1$ declines and increased albuterol use despite use of daily ICS controller therapy (**Fig. 5**). In a subsequent placebo-controlled study, the association between within-subject uLTE$_4$ changes and albuterol usage was shown to be blunted with LTRA use,

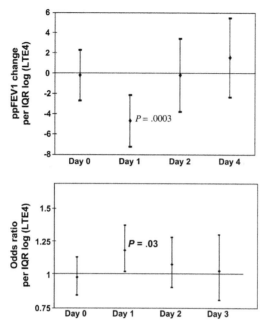

Fig. 5. uLTE$_4$ levels are associated with FEV$_1$ declines and increased albuterol use. Shown are the mean group estimates and the 95% confidence intervals for the association between daily percent predicted FEV$_1$ (ppFEV$_1$; *upper panel*) and daily medication use (*lower panel*), and uLTE$_4$ (logarithmic) levels measured on the same day (day 0) and up to 3 days later (day 3). The estimates are plotted per interquartile (IQR) (25th–75th) change in log uLTE$_4$. (*From* Rabinovitch N, Zhang L, Gelfand EW. Urinary LTE$_4$ levels are associated with decreased pulmonary function in children with persistent airway obstruction. J Allergy Clin Immunol 2006;118:637; with permission.)

suggesting that uLTE$_4$-associated health effects were mediated by CysLTs and not by other products that covary with CysLT levels.[70]

Several studies have shown associations between uLTE$_4$ levels and acute asthma exacerbations.[71,72] Green and colleagues[71] followed 180 adults who had asthma requiring visits to emergency departments in 16 sites across the United States. uLTE$_4$ levels were increased during asthma exacerbations compared with levels obtained 2 weeks later. Rabinovitch and colleagues[73] reported that schoolchildren exposed to secondhand tobacco smoke (SHS) were 3.5 times more likely to require at least 1 urgent care (UC) visit during the school year. In this study, the level of uLTE$_4$ was strongly associated with risk of at least 1 UC or emergency department (ED) visit in children exposed to SHS. uLTE$_4$ levels at a cutoff level of 106 pg/mg (measured by mass spectrometry assay) produced a 100% positive predictive value and a 78% negative predictive value for risk of ED or UC visits in children exposed to SHS. In this study, uLTE$_4$ was the only marker able to predict risk for exacerbation in SHS-related asthma. These results suggest a distinct biologic phenotype in asthmatics exposed to tobacco smoke in which CysLTs seem to play a prominent role in asthma severity. This model is supported by randomized adult[74] and pediatric[70] studies that have reported greater sensitivity to LTRA therapy in patients exposed to secondary or primary tobacco smoke. Further studies in other cohorts are required to validate the predictive value of uLTE$_4$ as a marker of increased risk for exacerbation in tobacco smoke–related asthma.

uLTE$_4$ AS A MARKER OF LTRA SUSCEPTIBILITY

Heterogeneity of responses to pharmacotherapy in asthma is of great practical interest. Clinical guidelines recommend that steroid-naive children with mild to moderate persistent asthma should be started on STEP-2 therapy with a low dose ICS therapy such as low-dose fluticasone propionate (FP). Alternative choices for STEP-2 therapy include an LTRA such as montelukast. In a randomized crossover study, Szefler and colleagues[75] and Zeiger and colleagues[76] reported significant individual variability in response to STEP-2 therapy with low-dose FP or montelukast. FE$_{NO}$ levels were associated with significant FEV$_1$ and asthma control day (ACD) responses to FP and to a better FP than montelukast response. In contrast, uLTE$_4$ levels greater than 100 pg/mg (measured with immunoassay in purified urine) were 3.2 times as likely to show a significant ($\geq$7.5%) FEV$_1$ response to montelukast therapy compared with children with lower levels. Cai and colleagues[77] studied lung function responses to montelukast in 61 patients who had asthma and concluded that patients with uLTE$_4$ levels greater than 200 pg/mg (measured by immunoassay in unpurified urine) were 3.5 times more likely to respond to LTRAs compared with those with lower levels.

Rabinovitch and colleagues[70] reported that uLTE$_4$-related albuterol usage and response to montelukast was related to the ratio of uLTE$_4$ to FE$_{NO}$ (uLTE$_4$/ FE$_{NO}$). A subsequent post hoc analysis of the Szefler and colleagues[75] study data as well as data from a second NIH-sponsored randomized pediatric asthma controller trial reported that uLTE$_4$ levels were associated with responses to either low-dose FP or montelukast therapy, whereas uLTE$_4$/FE$_{NO}$ levels were associated with a better FEV$_1$ and ACD response to montelukast than FP therapy.[78] Of the children with a better ($\geq$5%) FEV$_1$ response to montelukast than FP therapy, 86% had uLTE$_4$/FE$_{NO}$ ratios at or greater than 4, suggesting that children with low uLTE$_4$/FE$_{NO}$ ratios are highly unlikely to respond preferentially to montelukast monotherapy. These biomarker patterns might suggest a model of biologic heterogeneity related to STEP-2 medications (**Fig. 6**). In this model, high FE$_{NO}$ levels, indicating allergic airway inflammation, are associated with a clinically significant response to ICS therapy and a better

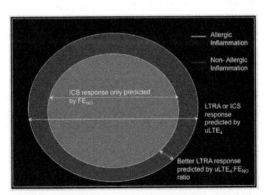

Fig. 6. Model of biomarker associations with STEP-2 therapy and related biologic phenotypes. High FE$_{NO}$ levels, indicating allergic airway inflammation, are associated with a clinically significant response to low-dose ICS therapy and a better ICS than LTRA response. In contrast, high uLTE$_4$ levels, indicating both allergic and nonallergic airway inflammation (as with cigarette smoke or ambient air pollution exposure), are associated with clinically significant responses to both ICS and LTRA therapy. High uLTE$_4$/FE$_{NO}$ ratios, indicating predominantly nonallergic airway inflammation largely resistant to ICS therapy, are associated with a better response to LTRA than to ICS therapy.

response to ICS than to LTRA therapy. In contrast, high uLTE$_4$ levels, indicating both allergic and nonallergic airway inflammation (as with cigarette smoke or ambient air pollution exposure), are associated with clinically significant responses to both ICS and LTRA therapy. As such, a high ratio of uLTE$_4$/FE$_{NO}$, indicating predominantly nonallergic airway inflammation largely resistant to ICS therapy, is associated with a better response to LTRA than to ICS therapy. Further prospective studies are required to test the sensitivity and specificity of these biomarkers to predict individualized responses to STEP-2 therapy.

SUMMARY

Measurement of uLTE$_4$ is a sensitive and noninvasive method of assaying total body CysLT production and changes in CysLT production. Recent studies have reported on novel LTE$_4$ receptor interactions, and new applications for uLTE$_4$, as a biomarker of environmental exposure to tobacco smoke and ambient air pollution, a predictor of risk for asthma exacerbations related to tobacco smoke, and a marker of susceptibility to leukotriene receptor antagonists.

ACKNOWLEDGMENTS

The author would like to thank Gretchen Hugen for assistance with preparation of the manuscript.

REFERENCES

1. Busse W, Kraft M. Cysteinyl leukotrienes in allergic inflammation: strategic target for therapy. Chest 2005;127:1312–26.
2. Lynch KR, O'Neill GP, Liu Q, et al. Characterization of the human cysteinyl leukotriene CysLT1 receptor. Nature 1999;399:789–93.
3. Evans J, Figueroa DJ. Cloning and expression of leukotriene receptors. Clin Exp Allerg Rev 2001;1:142–4.
4. Figueroa DJ, Breyer RM, Defoe SK, et al. Expression of the cysteinyl leukotriene 1 receptor in normal human lung and peripheral blood leukocytes. Am J Respir Crit Care Med 2001;163:226–33.
5. Mellor EA, Maekawa A, Austen KF, et al. Cysteinyl leukotriene receptor 1 is also a pyrimidinergic receptor and is expressed by human mast cells. Proc Natl Acad Sci U S A 2001;98:7964–9.
6. Woszczek G, Chen LY, Nagineni S, et al. IFN-gamma induces cysteinyl leukotriene receptor 2 expression and enhances the responsiveness of human endothelial cells to cysteinyl leukotrienes. J Immunol 2007;178:5262–70.
7. Pedersen KE, Bochner BS, Undem BJ. Cysteinyl leukotrienes induce P-selectin expression in human endothelial cells via a non-CysLT1 receptor-mediated mechanism. J Pharmacol Exp Ther 1997;281:655–62.
8. Datta YH, Romano M, Jacobson BC, et al. Peptido-leukotrienes are potent agonists of von Willebrand factor secretion and P-selectin surface expression in human umbilical vein endothelial cells. Circulation 1995;92:3304–11.
9. Hui Y, Cheng Y, Smalera I, et al. Directed vascular expression of human cysteinyl leukotriene 2 receptor modulates endothelial permeability and systemic blood pressure. Circulation 2004;110:3360–6.
10. Paruchuri S, Tashimo H, Feng C, et al. Leukotriene E4-induced pulmonary inflammation is mediated by the P2Y12 receptor. J Exp Med 2009;206:2543–55.

11. Volovitz B, Nathanson I, DeCastro G, et al. Relationship between leukotriene C4 and uteroglobulin-like protein in nasal and tracheobronchial mucosa of children. Implication in acute respiratory illnesses. Int Arch Allergy Appl Immunol 1988;86:420–5.

12. Heavey DJ, Soberman RJ, Lewis RA, et al. Critical consideration in the development of an assay for sulfidopeptide leukotrienes in plasma. Prostaglandins 1987; 33:693–708.

13. Tagari P, Rasmussen JB, Delorme D, et al. Comparison of urinary leukotriene E4 and 16-carboxyetranordihydroleukotriene E4 excretion in allergic asthmatics after inhaled allergen. Eicosanoids 1990;3:75–80.

14. Kumlin M, Dahlen B, Bjorck T, et al. Urinary excretion of leukotriene E4 and 11-dehydro-thromboxane B2 in response to bronchial provocation with allergen, aspirin, leukotriene D4 and histamine in asthmatics. Am Rev Respir Dis 1992;146:96–103.

15. Huber M, Muller J, Leier I, et al. Metabolism of cysteinyl leukotrienes in monkey and man. Eur J Biochem 1990;194:309–15.

16. Kumlin M, Stensvad F, Larsson L, et al. Validation and application of a new simple strategy for measurements of urinary leukotriene E4 in humans. Clin Exp Allergy 1995;25:467–79.

17. Kumlin M. Measurement of leukotrienes in humans. Am J Respir Crit Care Med 2000;161(2):S102–6.

18. Westcott JY, Maxey KM, Macdonald J, et al. Immunoaffinity resin for purification of urinary leukotriene E4. Prostaglandins Other Lipid Mediat 1998;55:301–21.

19. Armstrong M, Liu AH, Harbeck R, et al. Leukotriene-E4 in human urine: comparison of on-line purification and liquid chromatography-tandem mass spectrometry to affinity purification followed by enzyme immunoassay. J Chromatogr B Analyt Technol Biomed Life Sci 2009;1(877):3169–74.

20. Kishi N, Mano N, Asakawa N. Direct injection method for quantitation of endogenous leukotriene E4 in human urine by liquid chromatography/electrospray ionization tandem mass spectrometry with a column-switching technique. Anal Sci 2001;17:709–13.

21. Misso NL, Aggarwal S, Phelps S, et al. Urinary leukotriene E4 and 9a, 11b-prostaglandin F2 concentrations in mild, moderate and severe asthma, and in healthy subjects. Clin Exp Allergy 2004;34:624–31.

22. Kalayci O, Birben E, Sackesen C, et al. ALOX5 promoter genotype, asthma severity and LTC production by eosinophils. Allergy 2006;61:97–103.

23. Bizzintino JA, Khoo SK, Zhang G, et al. Leukotriene pathway polymorphisms are associated with altered cysteinyl leukotriene production in children with acute asthma. Prostaglandins Leukot Essent Fatty Acids 2009;81:9–15.

24. Di Lorenzo G, Pacor ML, Candore G, et al. Polymorphisms of cyclo-oxygenases and 5-lipo-oxygenase-activating protein are associated with chronic spontaneous urticaria and urinary leukotriene E4. Eur J Dermatol 2011;21:47–52.

25. Carry M, Korley V, Willerson JT, et al. Increased urinary leukotriene excretion in patients with cardiac ischemia. In vivo evidence for 5-lipoxygenase activation. Circulation 1992;85:230–6.

26. Hakonarson H, Thorvaldsson S, Helgadottir A, et al. Effects of a 5-lipoxygenase-activating protein inhibitor on biomarkers associated with risk of myocardial infarction: a randomized trial. JAMA 2005;293:2277–9.

27. Allen SP, Sampson AP, Piper PJ, et al. Enhanced excretion of urinary leukotriene E4 in coronary artery disease and after coronary artery bypass surgery. Coron Artery Dis 1993;4:899–904.

28. Hishinuma T, Suzuki N, Aiba S, et al. Increased urinary leukotriene E4 excretion in patients with atopic dermatitis. Br J Dermatol 2001;144:19–23.

29. Nakamura H, Hishinuma T, Suzuki N, et al. Difference in urinary 11-dehydro TXB2 and LTE4 excretion in patients with rheumatoid arthritis. Prostaglandins Leukot Essent Fatty Acids 2001;65:301–6.
30. Kim JH, Tagari P, Griffiths AM, et al. Levels of peptidoleukotriene E4 are elevated in active Crohn's disease. J Pediatr Gastroenterol Nutr 1995;20:403–7.
31. Simmet T, Luck W, Winking M, et al. Identification and characterization of cysteinyl-leukotriene formation in tissue slices from human intracranial tumors: evidence for their biosynthesis under in vivo conditions. J Neurochem 1990;54: 2091–9.
32. Sjostrom M, Johansson AS, Schroder O, et al. Dominant expression of the CysLT2 receptor accounts for calcium signaling by cysteinyl leukotrienes in human umbilical vein endothelial cells. Arterioscler Thromb Vasc Biol 2003;23:E37–41.
33. Gyllfors P, Kumlin M, Dahlén SE, et al. Relation between bronchial responsiveness to inhaled leukotriene D4 and markers of leukotriene biosynthesis. Thorax 2005;60:902–8.
34. Robbiani DF, Finch RA, Jaeger D, et al. The leukotriene C(4) transporter MRP1 regulates CCL19 (MIP-3beta, ELC)-dependent mobilization of dendritic cells to lymph nodes. Cell 2000;103:757–68.
35. Braccioni F, Dorman SC, O'Byrne PM, et al. The effect of cysteinyl leukotrienes on growth of eosinophil progenitors from peripheral blood and bone marrow of atopic subjects. J Allergy Clin Immunol 2002;110:96–101.
36. Kanwar S, Johnston B, Kubes P. Leukotriene C4/D4 induces P-selectin and sialyl Lewis (x)-dependent alterations in leukocyte kinetics in vivo. Circ Res 1995;77: 879–87.
37. Lee E, Robertson T, Smith J, et al. Leukotriene receptor antagonists and synthesis inhibitors reverse survival in eosinophils of asthmatic individuals. Am J Respir Crit Care Med 2000;161:1881–6.
38. Mellor EA, Austen KF, Boyce JA. Cysteinyl leukotrienes and uridine diphosphate induce cytokine generation by human mast cells through an interleukin 4-regulated pathway that is inhibited by leukotriene receptor antagonists. J Exp Med 2002;195:583–92.
39. Laitinen A, Lindquist A, Halme M, et al. Leukotriene E (4)-induced persistent eosinophilia and airway obstruction are reversed by zafirlukast in patients with asthma. J Allergy Clin Immunol 2005;115:259–65.
40. Bisgaard H, Olsson P, Bende M. Effect of leukotriene D4 on nasal mucosal blood flow, nasal airway resistance and nasal secretion in humans. Clin Allergy 1986;16:289–97.
41. Hay DW, Torphy TJ, Undem BJ. Cysteinyl leukotrienes in asthma: old mediators up to new tricks. Trends Pharmacol Sci 1995;16:304–9.
42. Espinosa K, Bossé Y, Stankova J, et al. CysLT1 receptor upregulation by TGF-beta and IL-13 is associated with bronchial smooth muscle cell proliferation in response to LTD4. J Allergy Clin Immunol 2003;111:1032–40.
43. Henderson WR Jr, Chiang GK, Tien YT, et al. Reversal of allergen-induced airway remodeling by CysLT1 receptor blockade. Am J Respir Crit Care Med 2006;173: 718–28.
44. Smith CM, Christie PE, Hawksworth RJ, et al. Urinary leukotriene E4 levels after allergen and exercise challenge in bronchial asthma. Am Rev Respir Dis 1991; 144:1411–3.
45. Hallstrand TS, Moody MW, Wurfel MM, et al. Inflammatory basis of exercise-induced bronchoconstriction. Am J Respir Crit Care Med 2005; 172:679–86.

46. Rabinovitch N, Silveira L, Gelfand EW, et al. The response of children with asthma to ambient particulate is modified by tobacco smoke exposure. Am J Respir Crit Care Med 2011;184:1350–7.
47. Rabinovitch N, Strand M, Gelfand EW. Particulate levels are associated with early asthma worsening in children with persistent disease. Am J Respir Crit Care Med 2006;173:1098–105.
48. Piedimonte G, Renzetti G, Auais A, et al. Leukotriene synthesis during respiratory syncytial virus bronchiolitis: influence of age and atopy. Pediatr Pulmonol 2005; 40:285–91.
49. Takahashi Y, Ichikawa M, Nawate M, et al. Clinical evaluation of urinary leukotriene e4 levels in children with respiratory syncytial virus infection. Arerugi 2003;52:1132–7.
50. Bisgaard H, Zielen S, Garcia-Garcia ML, et al. Montelukast reduces asthma exacerbations in 2 to 5 year-old children with intermittent asthma. Am J Respir Crit Care Med 2005;171:315–22.
51. Bartoli ML, Dente FL, Bancalari L, et al. Beclomethasone dipropionate blunts allergen-induced early increase in urinary LTE4. Eur J Clin Invest 2010;6:566–9.
52. Severien C, Artlich A, Jonas S, et al. Urinary excretion of leukotriene E4 and eosinophil protein X in children with atopic asthma. Eur Respir J 2000;16:588–92.
53. Mondino C, Ciabattoni G, Koch P, et al. Effects of inhaled corticosteroids on exhaled leukotrienes and prostanoids in asthmatic children. J Allergy Clin Immunol 2004;114:761–7.
54. Leigh R, Vethanayagam D, Yoshida M, et al. Effects of montelukast and budesonide on airway responses and airway inflammation in asthma. Am J Respir Crit Care Med 2002;166:1212–7.
55. Israel E, Rubin P, Kemp JP, et al. The effect of inhibition of 5-lipoxygenase by zileuton in mild-to-moderate asthma. Ann Intern Med 1993;119:1059–66.
56. Dahlen SE, Malmstrom K, Nizankowska E, et al. Improvement of aspirin-intolerant asthma by montelukast, a leukotriene antagonist: a randomized, double-blind, placebo-controlled trial. Am J Respir Crit Care Med 2002;165:9–14.
57. Overbeek SE, O'Sullivan S, Leman K, et al. Effect of montelukast compared with inhaled fluticasone on airway inflammation. Clin Exp Allergy 2004;34:1388–94.
58. Asano K, Lilly CM, O'Donnell WJ, et al. Diurnal variation of urinary leukotriene E4 and histamine excretion rates in normal subjects and patients with mild-to-moderate asthma. J Allergy Clin Immunol 1995;96:643–51.
59. Yamamoto H, Kuramitsu K, Houya I, et al. Clinical evaluation of urinary leukotriene E4 levels in asymptomatic bronchial asthma. Arerugi 1996;45:1106–11 [in Japanese].
60. Suzuki N, Hishinuma T, Abe F, et al. Difference in urinary LTE4 and 11-dehydro-TXB2 excretion in asthmatic patients. Prostaglandins Other Lipid Mediat 2000;62: 395–403.
61. Smith CM, Hawksworth RJ, Thien FC, et al. Urinary leukotriene E4 in bronchial asthma. Eur Respir J 1992;5:693–9.
62. Christie PE, Tagari P, Ford-Hutchinson AW, et al. Urinary LTE4 concentrations increase after aspirin challenge in aspirin-sensitive asthmatic subjects. Am Rev Respir Dis 1991;143:1025–9.
63. Oosaki R, Mizushima Y, Mita H, et al. Urinary leukotriene E4 and 11-dehydro-thromboxane B2 in patients with aspirin-sensitive asthma. Allergy 1997;52: 470–3.
64. Higashi N, Taniguchi M, Mita H, et al. Clinical features of asthmatic patients with increased urinary leukotriene E4 excretion (hyperleukotrienuria): involvement of

chronic hyperplastic rhinosinusitis with nasal polyposis. J Allergy Clin Immunol 2004;113:277–83.

65. Micheletto C, Visconti M, Tognella S, et al. Aspirin induced asthma (AIA) with nasal polyps has the highest basal LTE4 excretion: a study vs AIA without polyps, mild atopic asthma, and normal controls. Allerg Immunol (Paris) 2006;38:20–3.

66. Vachier I, Kumlin M, Dahlen SE, et al. High levels of urinary leukotriene E4 excretion in steroid treated patients with severe asthma. Respir Med 2003;97:1225–9.

67. Kurokawa K, Tanaka H, Tanaka S, et al. Circadian characteristics of urinary leukotriene E(4) in healthy subjects and nocturnal asthmatic patients. Chest 2001;120: 1822–8.

68. Bellia V, Bonanno A, Cibella F, et al. Urinary leukotriene E4 in the assessment of nocturnal asthma. J Allergy Clin Immunol 1996;97:735–41.

69. Rabinovitch N, Zhang L, Gelfand EW. Urine leukotriene E4 levels are associated with decreased pulmonary function in children with persistent airway obstruction. J Allergy Clin Immunol 2006;118:635–40.

70. Rabinovitch N, Strand M, Stuhlman K, et al. Exposure to tobacco smoke increases leukotriene E4-related albuterol usage and response to montelukast. J Allergy Clin Immunol 2008;121:1365–71.

71. Green SA, Malice MP, Tanaka W, et al. Increase in urinary leukotriene LTE4 levels in acute asthma: correlation with airflow limitation. Thorax 2004;59:100–4.

72. Oosaki R, Mizushima Y, Kawasaki A, et al. Urinary excretion of leukotriene E4 and 11-dehydrothromboxane B2 in patients with spontaneous asthma attacks. Int Arch Allergy Immunol 1997;114:373–8.

73. Rabinovitch N, Reisdorph N, Silveira L, et al. Urinary leukotriene E$_4$ levels identify children with tobacco smoke exposure at risk for asthma exacerbation. J Allergy Clin Immunol 2011;128:323–7.

74. Lazarus SC, Chinchilli VM, Rollings NJ, et al, National Heart Lung and Blood Institute's Asthma Clinical Research Network. Smoking affects response to inhaled corticosteroids or leukotriene receptor antagonists in asthma. Am J Respir Crit Care Med 2007;175:783–90.

75. Szefler SJ, Phillips BR, Martinez FD, et al. Characterization of within-subject responses to fluticasone and montelukast in childhood asthma. J Allergy Clin Immunol 2005;115:233–42.

76. Zeiger RS, Szefler SJ, Phillips BR, et al. Response profiles to fluticasone and montelukast in mild-to-moderate persistent childhood asthma. J Allergy Clin Immunol 2006;117:45–52.

77. Cai C, Yang J, Hu S, et al. Relationship between urinary cysteinyl leukotriene E4 levels and clinical response to antileukotriene treatment in patients with asthma. Lung 2007;185:105–12.

78. Rabinovitch N, Graber NJ, Chinchilli VM, et al, Childhood Asthma Research and Education Network of the National Heart, Lung, and Blood Institute. Urinary leukotriene E4/exhaled nitric oxide ratio and montelukast response in childhood asthma. J Allergy Clin Immunol 2010;126:545–51.

Index

Note: Page numbers of article titles are in **boldface** type.

A

Acetic acid, in exhaled breath condensate, 370–371
Acid reflux, exhaled breath condensate pH assays in, 382–383
Acidification, of airway. *See* pH assays, exhaled breath condensate.
Acute respiratory distress syndrome, exhaled breath condensate pH assays in, 382, 384
Aerocrine FENO monitoring system, 351–352
Age factors, in FENO values, 352
Airflow modeling, fractional concentration of exhaled nitric oxide and, 349–350
Albuterol, for asthma, 440
American Thoracic Society, FENO guidelines of, 349
Ammonia, in exhaled breath condensate, 370–371, 379–381
Asthma, biomarkers for
    bronchial hyperresponsiveness, **413–431**
    eosinophilic, 402–403
    exhaled breath condensate pH assays, 382, 384
    for remodeling, 406
    leukotriene E_4, 436–441
    neutrophilic, 404–405
    paucigranulocytic, 405–406
    sputum eosinophilia, **387–399**
Asthma Education Prevention Program, asthma definition of, 353

B

Biomarkers
    bronchoalveolar lavage-based, **401–411**
    exhaled breath condensate
        overview of, **363–375**
        pH assays, **377–386**
    exhaled nitric oxide, **347–362**
    for bronchial hyperresponsiveness, **413–431**
    in sputum, **387–399**
    tissue-based, **401–411**
    urinary leukotriene E_4, **433–445**
Breach condensate, exhaled. *See* Exhaled breath condensate.
Bronchial hyperresponsiveness, in asthma, **413–431**
    airway inflammation and, 416–417
    bronchoprovocation challenges for, 413–414, 418–423
    definition of, 413
    genetic component in, 414–415
    permanent components of, 415–416

Immunol Allergy Clin N Am 32 (2012) 447–451
http://dx.doi.org/10.1016/S0889-8561(12)00072-0
immunology.theclinics.com
0889-8561/12/$ – see front matter © 2012 Elsevier Inc. All rights reserved.

Bronchial (*continued*)
  therapy for, 417–418
  transient components of, 415–416
Bronchiolitis obliterans, FENO in, 356
Bronchoalveolar lavage-based biomarkers, in asthma, **401–411**
Bronchoprovocation challenges, in asthma, 413–414, 418–423
Bronchopulmonary dysplasia, exhaled breath condensate pH assays in, 382

C

Carbon dioxide, in exhaled breath condensate pH assays, 378
Chronic obstructive pulmonary disease
  exhaled breath condensate pH assays in, 382, 384
  FENO in, 354–355
Ciliary dyskinesia, primary, FENO in, 356
Corticosteroids
  FENO values and, 351–352
  for asthma, 392–396, 417–418, 437, 440–441
Cysteinyl leukotriene, biomarker for. *See* Leukotriene E$_4$.
Cystic fibrosis
  exhaled breath condensate pH assays in, 382
  FENO in, 355
Cytokines, in exhaled breath condensate, 371–372

D

Decorin, in asthma, 406

E

Enzyme immunoassays, for leukotriene E$_4$, 435
Eosinophilia, sputum, in asthma, **387–399**
Eosinophilic asthma, biomarkers for, 402–403
Eosinophilic inflammation, FENO values in, 351
Eotaxins, in asthma, 402–403
Ethyl alcohol, exhaled breath condensate pH assay interference from, 380
European Respiratory Society, FENO guidelines of, 349
Exhaled breath condensate, **363–375**
  biomarkers in
    future of, 373
    interpretation of, 372–373
    range of, 370–372
    source of, 364
  collection of, 366, 368–370
  contributors to, 363–364
  dilution of, 365
  for pH assays, **377–386**
  lack of gold standards for, 365–366
  oropharyngeal contribution to, 364–365
  particle size in, 364
  validation of, 366–367
Exhaled nitric oxide. *See* Fractional concentration of exhaled nitric oxide.

F

FENO. *See* Fractional concentration of exhaled nitric oxide.
Forced expiratory volume in one second, in asthma, versus sputum eosinophilia, 388–396
Formic acid, in exhaled breath condensate, 370–371
Fractional concentration of exhaled nitric oxide, **347–362**
    biology of, 347–349
    clinical use of, 352–356
    factors affecting, 351–352
    for airflow modeling, 349–350
    interpretation of, 349
    measurement of, 349
    normal values for, 350–351

G

Gastroesophageal reflux, exhaled breath condensate pH assays in, 382–383
Gender, FENO values and, 352
Genetic factors, in bronchial hyperresponsiveness, 414–415
Glucocorticoids. *See* Corticosteroids.

H

Histamine, in bronchial hyperresponsiveness, 414, 417
Histamine challenge tests, for asthma, 418–423
15-Hydroxyeicosetetrenoic acid, in asthma, 402–403

I

Immunoglobulin E, in bronchial hyperresponsiveness, 414
Interleukins
    in asthma, 402–403, 405
    in bronchial hyperresponsiveness, 415–417
    inhibitors of, for asthma, 418, 436–437, 440–441
Interstitial lung disease, FENO in, 355–356

L

Leukotriene(s)
    in asthma, 402–403, 405
    modifiers of, for asthma, 417–418
Leukotriene E_4, **433–445**
    as disease biomarker, 436–441
    measurement of, 435
    receptors for, 434–435
    synthesis of, 433
    variability of, 435–436
Lipooxygenase, in asthma, 402, 433
Liquid chromatography, for leukotriene E_4, 435
Lumican, in asthma, 406

M

Mannitol dry powder test, for asthma, 420–424
Mass spectrometry, for leukotriene E_4, 435
Mast cells, in asthma, 402
Matrix metalloproteinases, in asthma, 402, 405
Mechanical ventilation, exhaled breath condensate collection during, 368–370, 382
Methacholine challenge tests, for asthma, 418–423
Montelukast, for asthma, 440

N

Neutrophilic asthma, biomarkers for, 404–405
Nitric oxide, exhaled. *See* Fractional concentration of exhaled nitric oxide.

O

Oral collection, of exhaled breath condensate, 366, 368–369

P

Paucigranulocytic asthma, biomarkers for, 405–406
Pediatric patients, asthma in, sputum eosinophilia in, 390–392
pH assays, exhaled breath condensate, **377–386**
    carbon dioxide artifact in, 378
    clinical utility of, 381–384
    continuous monitoring in, 382
    determinants of, 380–381
    normal values for, 380
    probes for, 380
    research on, 381–384
    technical issues in, 378–380
    validation of, 378–380
Primary ciliary dyskinesia, FENO in, 356
Procollagen, in asthma, 406

R

Remodeling, in asthma, biomarkers for, 406
Respiratory infections, FENO values in, 352

S

Sarcoidosis, FENO in, 355–356
Scleroderma, FENO in, 355
Smoking, FENO values in, 352, 354–355
Sputum eosinophilia, in asthma, **387–399**
    corticosteroid effects on, 392–396
    in diagnosis, 388–389
    in management, 396–397
    in pediatric patients, 390–392

predicting relapse, 394–395
severity and, 389–391
STEP-2 therapy, for asthma, 440–441

T

Tenascin, in asthma, 402, 406
Tissue-based biomarkers, in asthma, **401–411**
Transforming growth factor-β, in asthma, 406
Tumor necrosis factor, in bronchial hyperresponsiveness, 416–417

U

Urinary leukotriene E$_4$. *See* Leukotriene E$_4$.

Z

Zileuton, for asthma, 437

Moving?

Make sure your subscription moves with you!

To notify us of your new address, find your **Clinics Account Number** (located on your mailing label above your name), and contact customer service at:

Email: journalscustomerservice-usa@elsevier.com

800-654-2452 (subscribers in the U.S. & Canada)
314-447-8871 (subscribers outside of the U.S. & Canada)

Fax number: 314-447-8029

Elsevier Health Sciences Division
Subscription Customer Service
3251 Riverport Lane
Maryland Heights, MO 63043

*To ensure uninterrupted delivery of your subscription, please notify us at least 4 weeks in advance of move.

Printed and bound by CPI Group (UK) Ltd, Croydon, CR0 4YY

03/10/2024

01040443-0013